1 MONTH OF
FREE
READING

at
www.ForgottenBooks.com

By purchasing this book you are eligible for one month membership to ForgottenBooks.com, giving you unlimited access to our entire collection of over 1,000,000 titles via our web site and mobile apps.

To claim your free month visit:
www.forgottenbooks.com/free864286

English
Français
Deutsche
Italiano
Español
Português

www.forgottenbooks.com

Mythology Photography **Fiction**
Fishing Christianity **Art** Cooking
Essays Buddhism Freemasonry
Medicine **Biology** Music **Ancient
Egypt** Evolution Carpentry Physics
Dance Geology **Mathematics** Fitness
Shakespeare **Folklore** Yoga Marketing
Confidence Immortality Biographies
Poetry **Psychology** Witchcraft
Electronics Chemistry History **Law**
Accounting **Philosophy** Anthropology
Alchemy Drama Quantum Mechanics
Atheism Sexual Health **Ancient History**
Entrepreneurship Languages Sport
Paleontology Needlework Islam
Metaphysics Investment Archaeology
Parenting Statistics Criminology
Motivational

THE RELATION

OF

ALIMENTATION AND DISEASE.

BY

J. H. SALISBURY, A. M., M. D., LL. D.

MEMBER OF THE PHILOSOPHICAL SOCIETY OF GREAT BRITAIN; MEMBER OF THE AMERICAN
ANTIQUARIAN SOCIETY; VICE-PRESIDENT OF THE WESTERN RESERVE HISTORICAL
SOCIETY; CORRESPONDING MEMBER OF THE NATURAL HISTORY SOCIETY
OF MONTREAL; MEMBER OF THE ALBANY INSTITUTE; MEMBER OF
THE AMERICAN ASSOCIATION FOR THE ADVANCEMENT OF
SCIENCE, ETC., ETC., ETC.

*Author of the Prize Essay on the Anatomy of Plants; of the Prize Essay on the Physiology and
Chemistry of the Maize Plant in its Various Stages of Growth; The Microscopic Examinations
of Blood and Vegetations found in Variola, Vaccina and Typhoid Fever; Malaria and
Vegetations of; Infusorial Catarrh and Asthma; Trichosis Felinis and Caninis; Cause
and Treatment of Diphtheria; Structure and Functions of the Spleen and Mesenteric
and Lymphatic Glands; Vegetations Producing Syphilis and Gonorrhœa; Vegetation in the Blood of Erysipelas; The Pus Cell an Infected Cell; Influence of the
Position of the Body on the Heart's Action; Diet and Drinks in Consumption;
Diet and Drinks in Diabetes; Diet and Drinks in Bright's Disease; Diet
and Drinks in Uterine Fibroids, Ovarian Tumors, Goitre, Fibrous
Growths generally, Locomotor Ataxy, and Rheumatism; Diet and
Drinks in Obesity; The Various Forms of Asthma and their Causes
and Treatment; Cause of Measles; Cause of Small Pox; Cause
of Typhoid Fever; Source of the Steatozoon Folliculorum;
Cause of Tubercular and Fibrous Consumption and
Consumption of Bowels and their Treatment;
Unhealthy Alimentation the Primary Cause of
all Diseases, aside from those Produced
by Injuries, Infections, and Poisons;
etc., etc., etc.*

SECOND EDITION

NEW YORK:
1892.

PREFACE.

In offering to the Medical Profession some of the results of over thirty years' research into the true Causes of Disease, a few words concerning the beginning and progress of my life-work will not appear misplaced.

In 1849 I began the study of germ diseases. Those of plants first occupied my attention; afterwards those in animals and in man. I had previously been engaged in the exact sciences of chemistry, botany, geology, zoölogy and mineralogy. In 1846 I was appointed assistant in the Chemical Laboratory of the New York State Geological Survey, and in 1849 I became Principal of the Laboratory. I had been a graduate of Albany Medical College, and in 1850 I entered upon the practice of medicine.

I was immediately and forcibly struck by the almost entire want of medical knowledge in regard to the true Causes of Disease, and by the consequent uncertainty that must and did exist as to the means of combating and curing pathological states. This uncertainty hampered me at each step of my practice. The art of Therapeutics was a chaos whose sole order consisted in dealing with established pathological conditions as though they were the disease itself, rather than what they actually were, viz.: consequences based upon antecedent and obscure states arising from an unknown Cause. In Consumption, for example, this want of thorough and basic knowledge conduced to our treating certain abnormal states as inflammatory, when they were in reality paralytic ones, as I shall demonstrate in subsequent pages.

The grim list of so-called " incurable diseases," and their steadily increasing death rates, riveted my attention and fascinated my thought. I attained an entire conviction that they must be curable; that since abnormal conditions could be established in previously healthy organisms, their causation must be discoverable, and that the mind of man must be endowed with sufficient power to trace the interlinked sequences of disease back to their primary source. I determined to accomplish this discovery, if possible, before my exit from this world. I started in without theories, without prejudices. I had no beaten rut to confine me. I resolved to collect and sift actual facts: to the ultimate testimony of these alone I looked for a solution of the riddle. Being a thorough microscopist and chemist, I began to make most searching examinations of every element of the human body — in health and in disease, — both microscopically and chemically. I made detailed drawings of every form met with, noting in connection with each drawing all of the conditions, states and symptoms found present in each. This work comprised microscopic examinations and drawings of blood; passages from bowels; deposits in urine; condition of and germs found in epithelium and mucus and mucous tissues; sweat; secretions from glands and follicles of the eye and other organs; the contents of the hair and fat follicles, and the condition of the ceruminous secretions. All this material was carefully filed away until enough should be accumulated in each disease to furnish its own history, and begin to throw some rays of light upon the dark picture.

In connection with this microscopic investigation I analyzed closely all parts of the human body, and also all the foods which were in constant use. This labor was persevered in until 1854, seemingly without resulting in much that was of real utility in handling disease with satisfaction to myself. These first five years of my medical experience were very laborious, anxious and painful ones to me, for I had started in to discover the primary Causes of pathological conditions in the human subject as revealed by complete evidence, and nothing less could satisfy my unalterable conviction.

In 1854 the idea came to me, in one of my solitary hours, to try the effects of living exclusively upon one food at a time. This experiment I began upon myself alone at first. Fortunately, in our works on Physiology, beans are placed at the head of the list of foods as regards their nutrient qualities. On this account I opened this line of experiments with baked beans. I had not lived upon this food over three days before light began to break. I became very flatulent and constipated, head dizzy, ears ringing, limbs prickly, and was wholly unfitted for mental work. The microscopic examination of passages showed that the bean food did not digest; that it fermented and filled the digestive organs with yeast, carbon dioxide, alcohol and acetic acid ; that the sacs of legumen containing starch granules were insoluble in the digestive fluids, and consequently these fluids could not reach the starch until it had fermented, and liberated sufficient gas to explode the sacs. By this time the starch was too far changed into gas, alcohol and vinegar, to afford much nourishment to the body.

From this date until September, 1856, I subjected myself to testing upon my own person the effects of exclusive feeding upon several other foods in turn, as often as I could find time to do so. My eyes opened to the vast reach of the field before me. I had found a door standing ajar, through which I began to get glimmerings of light in the right direction.

In September, 1856, I hired six well and hearty men to come and live with me, as I myself would live, on baked beans. This experiment and its results are fully described further on. In 1857 I engaged four other well men to live with me upon oatmeal porridge solely for thirty days. That experiment is also given in detail hereafter. In 1858 I took nearly 2,000 hogs in separate lots and in different pens, so that I might test various modes of feeding them, and carry my experiments on to the death point, as could not be done with men. In order to be sure of all my data, I tended, fed and dissected them myself; it was not work that could be done with kid gloves on! These experiments also are fully given in subsequent pages. Later on I employed men from time to time to live with me on other kinds of food, one kind at a time: some of the results of such living are duly given under their proper headings. By 1858 I began to understand from what Cause all our diseases emanate, excepting those arising from injuries, poisons and infections, and to hope that the day was not far distant when I should be able to cure them.

While prosecuting my studies upon feeding on one food at a time, I was taking every opportunity to get at the true Causes of infectious diseases. I began the study of smallpox germs in 1850, and worked at it fifteen years before I allowed myself to say or publish anything upon the subject.[1] In 1862 I worked up the measles germ and its source.[2] In 1862–63 I devoted much time to the causes of intermittent and remittent fevers and tracing them to their source.[3] During this period I also gave considerable attention to the study and discovery of the germ which produces diphtheria, asthma, and so on.[4]

Having satisfied myself as to the Causation of Disease, my next step was to complete a therapeutic system which should meet the facts in the case and attain the end in view, — that of combating a pathological groundwork by removing its cause, and thus effecting a radical cure. The publication of this work in its entirety has been delayed over twenty years, in order that sufficient cures of so-called " incurable " maladies might place both discovery and method of treatment beyond all reasonable doubt. Hundreds of cures now attest to their utility, not alone in my own practice, but also in that of other physicians of high repute, both here and in England.

---

[1] See work on Blood and Vegetations in Smallpox and Typhoid Fever, 1868.
[2] See *American Journal Med. Science* for July and October, 1862.
[3] See *Révue Scientifique*, Paris, 1869, and *American Journal Med. Science* for 1866.
[4] Gaillard's *Med. Journal*, New York, 1882.

In so far as the history of Consumption, in all its phases, is concerned, I do not at this juncture propose to do more than file a caveat, and give a clear outline of the Cause, development and cure of the disease. The result of my labors is given at some length in the ensuing chapters, together with other matter to be also more amply elaborated as time may serve. Medical terminology has somewhat changed since the writing of this work, but it is deemed best to leave this as it stood at the date of writing. The medical graduate of to-day will still have no difficulty in understanding these terms, and it is to him and to his comrades that this book is especially dedicated, in the hope that through its means the solicitude which clouded the outset of my career may be removed from theirs.

NEW YORK, March, 1888.

CONTENTS.

INTRODUCTORY REMARKS.

BEFORE treating of the pathological states and conditions of consumption and other diseases, and as a preliminary to the description of their physiological sequences, I shall briefly touch upon their original and underlying cause. Succinctly stated, this cause consists in pathological appetites and desires.

Appetites and desires are either physiological or pathological. They are the spontaneous yearnings of healthy states, or the cravings of diseased ones. Physiological appetites and desires presuppose a healthy organization. Pathological wants and longings are the outward manifestations of diseased organisms. Healthy intellectual and spiritual states are developed only in healthy conditions of the human system, while disordered mental efforts and moral fanaticisms are the outcrops of more or less deranged minds, which are themselves outward expressions of diseased states of the body.

Physical wants and animal passions are the yearnings of health or the cravings of disease. In perfect health, those foods only are desired that are best adapted to maintaining the system in a healthy condition.

Perfect health develops none but healthy physiological longings. Derange the human machine, either by physical, mental or moral disturbances, and pathological appetites, desires, cravings and hallucinations are the result. One step in the wrong direction opens the way for the second, the third and so on, till the human organism soon falls a victim to the disturbances of a multitude of deranging influences that result — if long continued — in fixed pathological habits of organs and tissues.

Surrounding relations, associations, circumstances, necessities, customs and fashions gradually develop morbid tastes within the healthy organism.

These tastes, regularly indulged in, become by degrees confirmed but cultivated abnormal habits; at the same time they derange organs and tissues little by little, until they result in pathological states.

When these physical derangements become firmly fixed, chronic disease of some kind is the result, its nature being determined by the character of, and long continuance in the gratification of specific unhealthy desires and appetites.

When the organs and tissues — either in function or structure, or in both — have become moulded to these morbidly deranged tastes and desires, the diseased states are thoroughly confirmed, and we have a well established chronic malady, which can now only be removed by removing or stopping its cause. This requires time, patience, resolution and a thorough determination on the part of the sufferer to get well.

It may safely be affirmed that all chronic diseases which afflict the human organism, aside from those arising from injuries, poisons and infections, have their genesis and development in something we are doing every day; or at least, in something to which we expose ourselves at regular and frequently repeated intervals. Occasional transgressions seldom or never result in confirmed pathological habits. Hence we must look to those states, conditions, acts, and things to which we are frequently, continuously and at fairly regular intervals exposed, to find the causes of nearly all our chronic ailments.

These various occurrences include drinks and foods; the kind, condition and proportions of each used; the state and rapidity with which they are taken in; the intervals at which they are drunk and eaten, and the quantities of each consumed. Also the nature and amount of labor and recreation; the amount of sleep, and the intervals and time at which it is taken; exposures to the various meteorological changes and conditions and the circumstances attending such exposures ; the frequency and kind of bathing ; the character of the clothing ; the nature and degree of mental, moral and physical excitements, the satisfaction of physical wants and animal passions and, in short, all the necessities, gratifications and events which sum up the doings of a human life.

THE RELATION OF ALIMENTATION AND DISEASE.

I.

USELESS EXPENDITURE OF NERVE FORCE IN INEFFECTUAL MENTAL EFFORTS.

THE two great factors of healthy organic life may be said to be : —

1st. Alimentation.

2d. Nerve Force, or Vital Energy.

Improper alimentation is the predisposing cause of disease.

Improper expenditure of nerve force hastens and assists in the maintenance of unhealthy states. Hence the judicious distribution and economical use of nerve force, becomes of the utmost importance in reëstablishing normal conditions.

Few persons are aware of the great amount of life force that is absolutely thrown away, which force is required to keep up the healthy actions of the organs of human life, — those organs through and by which we live, breathe and continue our existence in the body. This nerve force is unnecessarily expended in an almost constant and ineffectual working, day and night, of the faculties of the cerebrum ; a working without definite object or result, which the individual, apparently, has neither power nor knowledge to control. This thinking, feeling and worrying is under the influence and guidance of the emotional or sympathetic nerves, which are then really insane, or working wildly. Will-power, or voluntary mental effort, affords neither a balance-wheel nor a safety-valve to check this waste. The more the will-power, pure and simple, is brought to bear as a controlling and checking means, the greater the expenditure of nerve force.

This tendency and condition is always the outward expression of diseased states of the body. To control and check this waste we must get away from its cause, as far as is possible, and bring into operation healthy mental efforts. If these are persisted in, those faculties which are wildly working soon quiet down and the whole mental sphere becomes passive: this allows the nerve force to pass to the cerebellum and spinal ganglia — the nerve system of organic life. Then the machine, which before was either almost at a standstill or all out of balance, begins to run in a more normal manner, and a feeling of comfort and composure thrills through the entire mental and physical man.

The nerves of the senses of sight, hearing and touch, all have their origin in and near the cerebellum. By bringing these senses, or any one of them, into persistent operation for ten or more minutes, we can direct the nerve force to the cerebellum and establish it there. Then the stomach, bowels, diaphragm, heart, lungs and urinary and portal systems begin to receive sufficient vitality (through the distribution of the cerebellum) to set them in healthy action, and ere we are aware of it, the entire organism is calmly and passively working.

A variety of simple means may be resorted to in order to bring about this desirable change in the direction of expenditure of nerve force. All such means tend to calm the distracted, wildly acting faculties, and to set in motion healthy operations.

One easy and effectual plan is to get off alone, in a quiet room, where there is no noise nor other disturbing influence. The patient should be seated in an easy-chair, or lie upon a bed or lounge. The right hand should be placed with the palm on the forehead, and the palm of the left hand over the cerebellum and back of the neck. The eyes should be fixed upon some small object and persistently kept there: the breathings, which should be full, easy and slow, should be counted up to forty-nine, the patient all the time listening intently, as if expecting to hear something to advantage. When forty-nine inspirations have been reached, remove the right hand down to the pit of the stomach and the left hand to the opposite part of the back; now go through the operations previously suggested, when the hands were on the forehead and back of neck. When forty-nine inspirations are again reached, remove the right hand down over the umbilicus and the left hand to the small of the back, repeating all the operations as before. If they have been properly and quiescently conducted, the patient will either be happily sleeping or happy awake, before the last forty-ninth inhalation has been reached.

The rationale of this process is as follows. The palm of the right hand and the fore part of the body are both + (or positive) magnetic poles. The left palm and the back part of the body are both — (or negative) poles. Like poles repel, and by thus placing the palms of the hands over the various nervous centres or plexuses, a vital current is directed back into the body, its normal circuit is reëstablished, and its energies are guided and evenly distributed among the organs situate along its course. The physical and mental systems will become passive, contented, and comfortable, all parts working together for the common good. The result will be composure and recuperation. All distracting, harassing, melancholy imaginings and gloomy forebodings will have passed away; the stomach and bowels, and all their glandular appendages, will renew their healthy functions, while digestion and assimilation, previously at a standstill, will go on normally, producing a comfortable, delicious feeling throughout the entire system.

The method here suggested is only one of many which the good judgment of either physician or patient may devise, the object being simply to call in the scattered nerve forces, which are being wasted, and to transfer them to organs where they may be economically and usefully expended in the running of an enervated, unnerved, and more or less diseased organism.

The cerebrum almost uniformly uses up more of the nerve forces than the common good would entitle it to. It becomes often, — far too often, — in time and out of time, an extravagant user of nerve vitality, and all to no purpose; such workings are in the main, scattered, imaginary, wild and full of troubled shadows. This kind of mental operation belongs to the earliest pages of what may become, if long enough continued, a history of a case of insanity.

The cerebrum should not be permitted to work and consume vitality for more than ten hours in the twenty-four, on an average. The other fourteen hours should be spent in recreation, eating and refreshing sleep. If the organs and tissues are all in good order, and the diet, drinks and exercise what they should be, the cerebrum will become quiescent and rest wholly during sleep; the sleep will be refreshing and free from unpleasant dreams, while the nerve force will expend itself through the cerebellum and spinal ganglia in operating healthfully those organs over which we have little or no control.

When the cerebrum works abnormally, extravagantly scattering nerve force in every direction, the stomach and bowels halt, digestion and assimilation are seriously impaired, the food begins to ferment and decay, and peristaltic action is reversed, working the bile up into the stomach and back into the gall bladder, thus producing biliousness, which results in high-colored, scanty urine, dullness, lassitude and often headache.

So soon as the nerve forces are called in and turned into channels where they are needed, normal peristaltic action is restored, healthy digestion and assimilation begin, and headache and all other abnormal symptoms disappear.

We are all of us, especially the sick and debilitated, inclined to live and to expend nerve force too much in the cerebrum. We should strive to live more in the cerebellum and spinal ganglia, or, in other words, in the digestive apparatus and in the other vital organs which are run by the involuntary nerves. We should live less in the garret of our house and more in the kitchen. Our machines would then be kept in better repair, in better running order, and we should have a healthier organism, through which to expend our efforts in the accomplishment of good, useful and learned labors.

All healthy physiological actions, and all unobstructed normal tendencies in disease and health, move from the head towards the feet. When this progress is reversed, serious states and conditions manifest themselves, and unless the normal downward tendency is restored, there is danger ahead. All infections, fevers, colds, catarrhs, etc., begin at the head and progress gradually downward, taking their leave at the feet. When this natural course is interrupted or interfered with, so that its action is reversed, congestions and dangerous complications often ensue in the air passages, throat and head. Epilepsy represents an extreme and explosive reversed action in the nervous system : nervousness and wakefulness follow a mere tendency to reversed action therein. Biliousness and vomiting are the outcome of reversed peristaltic action in the digestive apparatus, and thus the vital energies are continually wasted, continually impeding organic action, through the useless friction of a possessed cerebrum.

Towards the close of this work I shall consider the possibility of increasing and storing vital force as a remedial means embraced in my plan of treatment. Meantime it can be quite as lavishly misused in physical as in mental operations; to the former I now call attention, while premising that this latter branch of the subject is the most neglected and the least understood.

II.

USELESS EXPENDITURE OF NERVE FORCE OR VITAL ENERGY, IN WASTEFUL, AIMLESS AND UNPROFITABLE PHYSICAL OPERATIONS.

A LIMITED amount of vital energy is given us, as a stock in trade, to carry us through this life, and while under ordinary circumstances, and in usual states and conditions, we can do but little to add to it, we can waste it lavishly in aimless and unprofitable operations, or in acts and exertions that have no enjoyable or valuable outcome.

Every pound of energy should be utilized and applied, when expended, to acts that shall result in usefulness or pleasure. Nothing should be thrown away, or cast aside into the waste basket. All exertion can be made to render its equivalent in good and advantageous results. All physical efforts should be made in the direction of recreation, enjoyment, profit and utility to ourselves and others. Our souls should be in every endeavor ; then we neither tire nor exhaust ourselves. When we are passive, interested machines for the accomplishment of useful and pleasurable ends and aims, we are in the inspirational and receptive state, where we can give or expend freely, and receive back freely in the same refreshing spirit. This state is that of great deeds, great exertions, great endurance and great results, without loss to the operator. The expenditure of energy in this passive, agreeable manner, leaves us as strong and fresh as we were before parting with it, if not more so. This is because, while in this state, we receive as much and often more than we give out. Under these circumstances and states, effort does not use us up and shorten life, but tends to strengthen and prolong it. On the contrary, all physical efforts that are entered into mechanically, unattended by that feeling of enjoyment and interest which makes a recreation of our work, are exhausting. They are consumers of vital energy, frequently closing up all the approaches through which the system receives an equivalent in return for expenditures. Such efforts, under such conditions, are constant and persistent drains on that given store of vital energy which each man possesses. This is illustrated in a marked degree by the professional gymnast, athlete, pugilist, oarsman, and so on. These men are much of the time on a mechanical treadmill drill in order to develop their muscles for greater feats of agility and endurance than they were originally intended to perform. The result is that their stock in trade of vital energy is, to a great extent, expended early in life; they become unable to engage longer in their profession, and in fact, die prematurely from a lack of that vitality without which they cannot longer survive. They are usually worn out at from thirty-five to forty, and die from forty-five to fifty-five. These are extreme illustrations of lavish expenditure of life principle; of vital energy thrown recklessly away. Such persons are mere curiosities of existence, of no use save to demonstrate some of life's follies and short-sightedness. A large class of the community are, in less degree, steadily expending their vital energies in the same aimless manner. Baseball playing, boxing, health-lift exercises, and all other physical efforts of this character that make labor-machines of us, result in throwing away priceless energy, which, if stored up, might prolong our lives and enhance their humanitarian value. Everywhere, at all times and in all places, we should be constant economists, using judgment and discretion in the expenditure of vital energy, both in mental and in physical operations. When living this passive, inner life, actuated by feeling and the interior impressions, we soon find these subjective forces expressing themselves in the outer life by a correlated and healthy activity. Passive to the higher sphere of Thought, and wisely active to that of the objective world; receptive of noble impulse and distributive of true deeds, we become a living magnet with its poles ; a great current of power flows into us and from us ; we do not dam up the stream nor yet dribble it ignorantly away. We enter into all operations with a love and faith which make our efforts a joy and not a trial, and without fatigue, as without conscious strain, we receive an equivalent for the life force we expend. " Freely give, freely receive." This is the secret of living long and living well. If we could keep ourselves in the passive, receptive, inspirational state, we should always be receiving as freely as we bestow, and we should be permitted to live on and on, without much wear and tear, retaining health and vigor far along in years, and no one knows to what age the mortal body might not be made a comfortable and suitable dwelling-place for the immortal. Generations of mistaken education have made us a race of outside livers. We live and act almost entirely from appearances and not from realities. For the accomplishment of some selfish, underhanded, or ambitious end, we are forever putting on fictitious semblances to cover up the devious routes by which we expect to arrive, in our own way, at results which we imagine will prove beneficial to ourselves. In consequence we find on looking over the ground of human action, that men see and reason from the delusive side, instead of from the real one. We have become surface and hypocritical thinkers, talkers, and doers : we live unnatural and exhausting lives, full of perversities, fluctuations, animosities, bewilderment and sin. No inspirational feeling ; no sincere soul work ; no abiding faith in the high rectitude of our Being : we exist, struggling on and on under this fearful depletion, until we experience the natural outcome of a misspent course and die amid our suffering. Our end comes prematurely, a miscarriage, a painful labor, and we are ushered to " the other side," to the immortal existence, in a perverted and unripe state, quite unfit for its beautiful harmonies and realities.

III.

ALIMENTATION.

ALIMENTATION may be classified under two heads, namely: Healthy Alimentation and Unhealthy Alimentation.

Healthy Alimentation is the feeding upon that or those kinds of food which any given animal organism is designed to live upon, as indicated by the structure and functions of its digestive apparatus.

Unhealthy Alimentation is the feeding upon food which the digestive organs cannot readily and perfectly digest. For instance, we should not for a moment think of feeding our cattle, horses and sheep upon lean and fat meats, neither do we expect to feed cats and dogs upon hay, corn and oats. If we should attempt any such digression, we should very soon have all these animals diseased, for this would constitute unhealthy alimentation, or the feeding upon food for which the digestive organs were not intended. That which would be healthy alimentation for horses, cattle and rabbits, would be unhealthy alimentation for the cat and dog, and vice versa. What would be healthy alimentation for purely herbivorous and purely carnivorous animals would be unhealthy alimentation for man, since he partakes structurally of both the herbivora and carnivora, and belongs to the omnivora.

Food productive of disease in the horse, ox and rabbit, might be healthy food for the dog and cat, while that which might induce disease in either the purely herbivorous or the purely carnivorous animals, might be healthy food for man and in him promote health. Hence it is evident that experiments performed with food upon the horse, ox or rabbit, cannot in their result be applied either to the dog and cat, or to man. In experimenting in this direction, each class must stand alone, and must be studied independently of all others.

By structure, man is about two-thirds carnivorous and one-third herbivorous. In his native, wild state he feeds mainly upon game and fish, with much less than one-third of vegetable products. In this state he is free from most of our fatal diseases, such as Consumption, Bright's Disease, Diabetes, Locomotor Ataxy, Paralysis, Fatty diseases of vital organs, Tumors, and the various forms of Cancer. He is also exempt from most infectious complaints, such as Smallpox, Measles, Scarlet Fever, Diphtheria, and so on. These only reach him when he comes in contact with our much lauded civilization — a civilization full of " shirking responsibility," of sin and of the causes of disease.

There are indeed individuals, as well as nations, who have made themselves herbivorous. Long generations of vegetarianism, and inherited organic tendencies have inured their systems to this mode of feeding. In such cases the stomach, or meat-digesting organ, has but little work to do; the pyloric valve is paralyzed and remains permanently open, and the vegetable food passes through the organism, being chiefly digested by the biliary secretions, the small bowels and their glandular appendages. Such persons have, as a rule, less nervous and muscular endurance than meat-eaters. Officers of the English army in India, for example, assure me that it is always necessary to start the native troops off on a march one day in advance of the British soldiers, that all may arrive at a given point on the same day.

In the wild state, death is seldom brought about by disease, but is usually the resultant of accident or of old age. The death rate in youth and middle age is comparatively small, accidents excepted. I have known many North American Indians of temperate habits, who were hale, hearty and straight as an arrow, when over one hundred years old. In 1860, I was called to see the wife of a prominent Indian chief, who was lying ill with pneumonia. She was one hundred and four years of age, while her husband was one hundred and six. He was erect and vigorous, appearing no older than a civilized man of sixty. Among the native, wild tribes of Central America many persons are found to be considerably over one hundred years of age. In one instance, where records have been kept, a man now living, active and in good health, is known to be over one hundred and fifty, and is supposed to be nearly two hundred years old.[1]

There is no reason why we of civilized communities should not live to an even greater age than man does in the wild state, if we would but avoid the causes of the fatal diseases previously enumerated. These causes are simple ones, and have their origin in our daily habits of living; in the cultivated tastes for unnatural nutriment, preparations and drinks, and in the various exposures to infections — cryptogamic and infusorial — developed in and by abnormal surroundings, states and conditions. All of these may be readily avoided if we will but read a few plain lessons from the book of Nature, ever open before us.

In infancy, we may avoid sickness, disease and death, by observing certain obvious indications. An infant is not a week old, before it is " dosed " almost perpetually with anise and " catnip " teas for its acid stomach, its severe colic pains, and vomiting sour and curdled milk. The child is not a day old before it is over and unnaturally fed. It is fed too frequently, too much at a time, and often with food that no infant stomach could digest. The natural food for an infant is the plain mother's milk. When this cannot be had, cow's or goat's milk may be substituted. Avoid all " panadas," cracker and sago preparations, sweetened milk and water, etc., etc. The child

---

[1] In Rio de Janeiro there is a Spanish physician — a meat-eater — who is now one hundred and ninety-three years of age, and who is yet quite strong and active, mentally and physically.

should be fed only a small quantity at a time; just what it can digest easily without undergoing alcoholic and acid fermentation, and at regular intervals of about three hours. If this course be taken, the child will be and continue free from pain and all dyspeptic trouble, and will thrive, sleep, eat and be happy.

This kind of feeding should be persevered in till Nature holds out the sign for the gradual introduction of lean meats into the dietetic list. This moment is indicated by the gradual development of the meat teeth. With the first appearance of the incisors, beef tea and the juice of beef may be introduced, and finally beefsteak and other lean meats may be partaken of with the milk. Starchy and other vegetable products and fruits should not enter the diet list until the vegetable teeth, or grinders, begin to show themselves.

By following these simple rules all colics, dyspeptic troubles, "summer complaints" and the attendant head complications may be avoided, and the consequent great fatalities, of childhood escaped.

During the period when the mother is carrying the child in utero, she should be careful to live upon plain, substantial food, eschewing all preparations that derange the digestive apparatus, thereby interfering with healthy digestion and assimilation. The diet should be about two parts of lean meats, either broiled or roasted, to one part of vegetable food and fruits. The fruit should be used sparingly, and only after breakfast or dinner. Exercise should be taken freely and daily in the open air, and all excitements, sudden surprises, severe work, and over-exertion should be avoided.

By pursuing this course through the period of gestation, parturition is made easy, and there is but little danger of abnormal conditions and floodings during and after labor. After birth, the mother should continue to live upon the substantial diet heretofore named, keeping it up throughout the entire nursing period, which should continue about twelve months. After weaning, cow's milk should take the place of mother's milk. As far as possible, this should be taken so soon as milked, while it is still warm and full of animal life and heat. In this condition it is readily digested and assimilated. The difference between milk alive and warm from the cow, and cold, dead milk, is fully understood by breeders of fine stock. They know well that a calf which is allowed to suckle its mother is more than three times the size — when a year old — than one of the same age and breed which has been fed on cold, dead milk. The one which sucks the warm, vital milk is large, robust, trim and elegant in shape, and vigorous in constitution, while the one which is fed on cold, dead milk is " pot-bellied," pointed at both ends, ungainly in shape, small, and has the appearance of belonging to an inferior breed.

This fact should impart a valuable lesson to those interested in rearing children, and by taking advantage of the stockbreeder's knowledge, show them how they may gradually develop a higher and more perfect physical and mental type of the human organism.

IV.

HEALTHY ALIMENTATION.

As a general rule, we have twenty meat teeth, and only twelve vegetable teeth ; while four of these latter, the " wisdom teeth," are poor apologies as grinders.   The stomach, in man, is a purely carnivorous organ, and is designed, both in structure and function, for the digestion of lean meats.   The small bowels, with their glandular appendages (liver, pancreas, and glands of Lieberkuhn and Brunner), are herbivorous mainly, and are designed to digest vegetables, fats and fruits.   The pancreatic secretions are used to emulsify fats, and to change starch into glucose.   The biliary secretions, and those of the glands of Lieberkuhn and Brunner, are for digesting farinaceous and vegetable products generally.   Healthy Alimentation would consist in a diet of about one part of vegetables, fats and fruits, to about two parts of lean meat.   Sweets and fruits should be used in moderate quantity, and as relishes only.   Fruits should only be taken after breakfast and dinner, on a full stomach, and then only in moderate quantity ; never at or after supper.   The supper should be more of a lean meat meal than either of the others, and the best meat for supper is broiled lean beef.   This digests easily and quickly, and is less liable to produce flatulence than any other food.

It is not enough to take solely into account the chemistry of foods.   Many foods which are chemically rich are so composed that it is beyond the power of human stomachs and bowels to digest them.   The connective tissue of meat, on the one hand, and beans on the other, are products that no human being should undertake to subsist upon ; if he does, he will expose himself to causes that imperil healthy states.

The bean is chiefly made up of double walled sacs of legumen, which are filled with starch grains. These sacs are as insoluble in the digestive fluids as woody fibre, and the only way in which the secretions of the digestive organs can get at the contents of these insoluble sacs, is by the starch grains undergoing fermentation. This liberates large quantities of carbonic acid gas, which gas explodes the sacs. By the time the digestive fluids reach the contents of these exploded sacs, the starch is decomposed into carbonic acid gas, alcohol, vinegar and yeast vegetation, products that are quite unfitted to afford healthy nourishment, but are rather agents to feed pathological states. By examining the stools with the microscope, the day after a diet of beans, the whole mass will be found to be made up of exploded and non-exploded sacs of legumen, and the products of their fermenting contents.

All vegetables and fruits have their starch and other nutritious products enclosed in single walled sacs of an albuminoid character. These are somewhat insoluble, so that it requires a healthy state of the digestive organs to dissolve their walls before the contents begin to ferment. They are, however, far more easily and expeditiously digested than beans.

The starch and other nutritious products of grains are not enclosed in sacs at all; hence the digestive fluids coming in contact with them as soon as eaten, renders them much more easily digested than vegetables.

These few remarks will be a guide to the selection of such vegetable foods as can be most readily digested in health or disease. When food only is eaten that digests and assimilates well, there is no fermentation or flatulence in the digestive organs, and the urine flows at the rate of from $3\frac{1}{2}$ to $4\frac{1}{2}$ pints daily, stands at a density of 1.015, and is free from sediment on standing in the cold. As soon as food that cannot be digested is taken, more or less flatulence occurs, which reverses to a greater or lesser extent normal peristaltic action. This works the bile up into the stomach, and back into the gall bladder and gall ducts ;   the patient becomes what is called " bilious," the urine is high colored and scanty, and stands at a density of 1.030 and upwards, and deposits a sediment on standing.

V.

UNHEALTHY ALIMENTATION A PRIMARY CAUSE OF DISEASE, AND HEALTHY ALIMENTATION A CURATIVE PROCESS.

HEALTHY alimentation, or feeding upon such foods as the system can well digest and assimilate, is always promotive of health. Unhealthy alimentation always acts as a cause of disease.

Special feeding, indicated by the condition of the system, acts as a means of cure in all diseases arising from unhealthy feeding. By special feeding in any disease is meant the living on precisely such food as can be most thoroughly digested and assimilated, or upon such food as the diseased tissues require, and upon no other. When living in this way the system is steadily and gradually getting into better order; the appetite improves; the urine becomes clear and of the proper density and quantity; the feces healthy in consistence and color; the skin moist and soft, and all the mucous surfaces are in a normal state.

Some of the diseases arising from unhealthy alimentation are as follows : Consumption, *in all its phases*, including " chronic diarrhœa " and summer complaints in children ; dyspepsia, in all its forms ; rheumatism, in all its varieties ; gout, Bright's disease, diabetes mellitus, locomotor ataxy, ovarian tumors, goitre and cretinism. All fibrous tumors, including uterine fibroids and cancerous growths. All paralytic diseases, except those arising from injuries, poisons and infections. Softening of the brain, and most cases of insanity which have not been produced by injuries, inflammations and effusions ; purpura hæmorrhagica ; all forms of deafness, and diseases of the eye and ear that have not resulted from injuries, poisons, exposures and infections ; all catarrhs, thickenings and fibrous diseases of the digestive organs and air passages (aside from those caused by injuries, poisons and infections); all forms of gravel of the urinary and biliary organs, and of the lungs; asthma in all its forms, except such as result from animal and vegetable parasites; all fatty diseases of the heart and other organs, excepting such as result from injuries; anæmia in its various forms; most cases of prolapsus of the bowels and uterus; many demented conditions; hypochondria; most cases of loss of voice; erysipelas; eczema; scald-head, etc., etc.

By unhealthy alimentation, then, is meant the too exclusive, too long-continued feeding upon any one kind of food. This species of feeding overtaxes those portions of the alimentary canal designed for digesting this particular character of aliment, and overtaxes them so far that the digestive process soon becomes imperfect and fermentation gradually supervenes.

The blood before long begins to show signs of deterioration, and the physiological processes of the various tissues depending upon good blood for their healthy support are gradually disturbed; hence pathological states of the histological elements arise by degrees. The normal processes of cell feeding, cell digestion, cell assimilation, cell organization and cell elimination all become more or less deranged and the various organs and tissues — being supplied with abnormal, imperfect material for carrying on their normal functions in a physiological manner — yield step by step to pathological invasion, and palpable disease soon results.

The abnormal states produced by a too exclusive amylaceous and saccharine diet, differ from those produced by one that is too exclusively carnivorous. The former present themselves where the diet is exclusive, highly fermentable and profuse, while the victim is leading an inactive or sedentary life, and present the following interlinked sequences.

A. Yeasty, gaseous, highly deranged, half paralyzed state of the alimentary canal and nervous system, conjointly with a marked tendency to fibrinous deposits as thrombi in the heart and large vessels leading to it.

B. These fibrinous deposits break loose from their fastenings and constitute emboli.

C. They float along the blood stream, and if too large to pass through the capillaries they are —

D. Liable to be caught up by these vessels in the lungs, mesentery and other organs, or in the extremities, there producing embolism.

When less exclusive and less excessive, this kind of feeding may not eventuate in thrombosis and embolism. But if long adhered to, it may partially paralyze the mucous surfaces of the digestive organs, when the following states are caused and ensue in the order set forth.

A. The mucous surfaces (especially in the stomach and large bowel) are made to secrete a thick, ropy, tenacious, gelatinous mucus.

B. This mucus clogs the follicles.

C. The obstruction — joined to the paralysis of the mucous surfaces of the digestive organs — produces a stasis of the parts, and causes —

D. Hypernutrition of the tissues named, and of the fibrous tissues around and beneath, under a state of partial death.

E. Consequent thickening of the walls, especially those of stomach and colon. If allowed to go on unhindered these states may further bring about —

F. Occlusion of the intestinal canal.

G. In some cases, also, the new tissue formed may become so hardened and poorly supplied with blood-vessels and nerves as to produce scirrhus.

In still other instances the fibrous or connective tissue may be excessively formed in one or both ovaries, together with an excessive secretion of the so-called colloid matter (gelatinous, ropy, viscid mucus) from the gland cells of these organs, forming a saccate growth of large size, — the so-called ovarian tumor.

In other cases, connective or glue tissue may begin to be excessively formed and deposited in the walls of, or attached to the inside or outside of the organ. This process may go on with greater or lesser rapidity — according to the excess in abnormal vegetable diet and state of the digestive organs — till the growth has acquired a very large size. Under certain influences this growth becomes hardened or cartilaginous, when scirrhus is the result.

In other instances, fibrous growth may take place in the tendons or fasciæ, or sheaths of organs or muscles in any part of the body, resulting in the various tumors, or the different types of excessive development of connective or glue tissue in places where it does not normally belong. In other instances, again, the fibrous sheaths of the nerves may thicken in certain localities, forming the so-called sclerosis. This may occur in the spinal cord, and results in progressive paralysis (locomotor ataxy) in the brain, producing demented and deranged conditions. Or it may occur in nerve sheaths in any part of the body, accompanied by more or less paralysis and numbness.

No matter where these excessive developments of glue tissue may occur, they all emanate from such fermentative changes in the alimentary canal as serve to generate poisonous, highly paralyzing gases and yeast products. These, in the first instance, partially paralyze the nerves of the part about to be affected; a stasis or dilated state of the vessels hence ensues. The blood then accumulates, and the connective and mucous tissues are often overfed, or glutted with food. The diseased parts grow with abnormal rapidity, but in most cases the new tissue is poorly supplied with nerves and blood-vessels, except when the growth attacks the sheaths of the blood-vessels; in this case the growth is excessively rapid and over-abundantly supplied with nerves and blood-vessels.

The point of attack, in any given case, is determined by the previous weakened state of the nerves and tissue of a given part. The weakest, most exposed, most abused and most used part or organ falls first a victim, because the operative influences bring such part or organ into a state fitted to take on diseased action. The disease proceeds along the line of least resistance. The basic step in the excessive development of connective tissue in any part, is thus seen to consist in the too exclusive feeding on fermentable, amylaceous and saccharine foods. This step is hastened by inactivity and the fermentation of these foods in the alimentary canal, developing large quantities of carbonic acid gas and alcoholic and acid yeasts. This fermentation prevents healthy digestion and assimilation, and soon the mucous surfaces become so paralyzed that they lose their normal selective power as displayed in health. These poisonous products and acid-forming plants then begin to be taken up, which ushers in the third step — that of partial paralysis of the parts about to be affected. This brings about a dilated state of the blood-vessels and a stasis in them, the outcome of which is a peculiar hypernutrition, by virtue of which connective or glue tissue and also epithelial tissue (where it is involved with the other) of a low type are formed in excess.

It is a wise and fortunate provision that nearly all excessive growths shall take place in the connective or glue tissues; in the bony and cartilaginous tissues, and in the epithelial and fatty tissues. By far the largest proportion occur in the connective tissue. All these tissues have a low grade of vitality, and have for their office the making up of a substantial framework supplied with all the necessary cords, bands, sheaths, coverings and upholsterings for protecting, supporting and enveloping the more highly vitalized tissues.

If we feed as nature designed us to do, all these tissues may be maintained in perfect health. They become diseased by our departures from the " strait and narrow path," in which we should travel gastronomically. We may look to the foods and fluids of civilized life for a large causal share in those " ills that flesh is heir to." The abnormal conditions herein set forth become simple systemic expressions, warning us against the further transgression of dietetic laws.

Thus the philosophy of this physiological work is to dispense with all foods, drinks and medicines which tend in any way whatsoever to getting and keeping the histological elements, organs and tissues out of order, and to persistently and continuously feed and starve tissue so long as any remnant of disease remains. Healthfully feeding those tissues which require nourishing, and starving such as have been over and unhealthily fed, will in time restore the equipoise of an unbalanced organism.

VI.

PREDISPOSITION TO CONSUMPTION.

IT is well established that some organizations are much more liable, under the same set of circumstances, to take on the consumptive disease than are certain others. This tendency exists from infancy. It indicates an abnormal systemic state, brought about — often — by generations of unhealthy feeding: it is produced by a well-defined cause. This cause may start in utero and continue in latent operation for a few months, or for a few, or for many, years after birth before the disease becomes well defined.

During all of this incubative period there is a well-marked cause insidiously operating. In most, if not in all cases, this cause may be determined by means of the microscope, taken in connection with the physical conformation and the condition of the organism.

The cause of this predisposition to consumption cannot be said to be hereditary, but may start from the food received by the fœtus in utero, from the mother's milk while nursing, or from the character of diet, surroundings and other accompanying conditions later in life.

Consumption often appears to run in families, many or all of their members dying with it, either early or at a more advanced age. This has led many investigators to suppose that the cause of the disease is transmissible from parents to children, or in other words, that it is hereditary.

Strictly speaking, this is not the case, as is shown by the fact that the disease may be developed in any person, no matter how robust and free from the supposed hereditary taint, by simply feeding them on special fermentable and fermenting foods, as will be shown further on.

The reason why consumption seems to be hereditary in certain families, is that all such families are in the habit of living too exclusively upon the fermentable foods which produce this disease. This kind of feeding, continued for several generations, develops a conformation of the chest and an organization of body and mind which render the system easily liable to take on the disease, under the influence of favoring diet and conditions. Most or all members of the same family are very apt to fall into the same habits of feeding : all are liable to feed (so to speak) "out of the same trough."

Of course we then find the same or similar diseases, arising from unhealthy alimentation, developing, as we might expect, in all the members of such families.

This is the reason why consumption has been supposed to be — as to the surface observer it seems — an hereditary disease, or one transmissible from parents to children ; a certain and necessary heirloom in families.

That it is not a hereditary disease, but one solely dependent upon alimentation and the states of the system developed by unhealthy feeding, is evidenced further by the fact that so-called consumptive children, when taken from consumptive families and put upon good, healthy alimentation in meat eating families, lose the tendency to the disease and become vigorous, healthy and free from all signs of consumption. Vice versa, children the most exempt and the least liable to it may be made its victims if fed too exclusively upon fermenting or fermentable foods when exposed to the proper conditions.

VII.

THE ORDER OF INVASION.

WHEN persons are put exclusively upon a farinaceous and saccharine diet, with plenty of sweet drinks and but little exercise, consumption of the bowels precedes that of the lungs, the disease attacking the large intestines before it has had time to reach the lungs through the circulation. Sooner or later, however, the lungs become involved, provided the patient survives.

When the fermenting food is somewhat mixed with lean meats, while there is yet not enough of the latter to keep the stomach active and in good condition, fermentative changes begin slowly in the stomach (especially if the patient be engaged in sedentary pursuits) and after a longer or shorter period, extend gradually to the small bowels. These surfaces become gradually paralyzed by the constant development and contact of carbonic acid gas, so that the products of fermentation begin to be taken up and pass into the circulation before the large bowels become involved. There is, then, danger of the pulmonary tissues becoming invaded before the large intestines are so, in which case pulmonary phthisis precedes consumption of the bowels.

Hence the order of invasion depends upon the kind and proportion of unhealthy alimentation.

VIII.

CONSUMPTION : ITS CAUSES AND DEVELOPMENT.

CONSUMPTION, strictly speaking, is a disease caused by abnormal or unhealthy feeding, or feeding too exclusively upon the various preparations of grains, vegetables, sweets and fruits, and the products developed from them by fermentation.

By structure, we are about two-thirds carnivorous, and one-third herbivorous, and if we wish to maintain the human machine in good running condition, we must expect to feed it upon the foods that it is made to digest well. Any continued and persistent departure from this rule, constitutes unhealthy alimentation, and is liable — except within certain moderate limits and under certain favorable conditions and circumstances — to result more or less rapidly in pathological disturbances. These are at first local, then more general, and finally terminate, soon or late, in well-defined diseases.

Consumption is a disease of this character, — one that is produced by certain and too exclusive feeding upon the various preparations of grains, vegetables, sweets and fruits, and the products developed by their fermentation. When fed too exclusively upon these fermentable foods, the overtaxed stomach and bowels are unable to digest them ; alcoholic and acetic fermentation set in, and the digestive apparatus is soon clogged with yeast vegetations and the enervating and poisonous products developed by their growth. If the diet is entirely, or almost entirely of a fermentable character, and but little exercise is taken, the stomach and bowels are soon so greatly disturbed with yeasty products that this yeast, from its bulky, irritating and paralyzing character, passes off in many stools daily. This constitutes consumption of the bowels.

If the diet be less exclusive, and the exercise sufficient to digest part of the food, the yeasty matters accumulate less rapidly, and the system being better able to resist their poisonous and irritating influences, the disease progresses more slowly. In consequence of this, the yeast plants and the products of their growth remain in the small intestines long enough to so paralyze the villi and mucous surfaces generally, that the cells lose their normal selective power; hence the spores of the mycoderms are gradually taken up and carried into the blood stream, where after a longer or a shorter period they so accumulate in elongated masses, or emboli, as to be too large to float through the capillary vessels of the lungs. At this stage tubercular deposits begin, and go on increasing as fast as the masses of yeast in the blood stream develop to the proper size.

IX.

CONSUMPTION AND ITS CAUSATIVE VEGETATIONS.

THE vegetations that act as causes of, and aggravating accessories to, consumption are the various alcoholic and acid yeasts.
The former belong to the genus Saccharomyces, and the latter to
the genus Mycoderma. The Saccharomyces develop in the
stomach and bowels, in the mouth, throat and fauces, and often
in the lungs during the later stages of the disease, and frequently
the entire epidermic surfaces of the body are filled with the
spores of this yeast vegetation.[1]

1 This book with all its illustrations was ready for the press in 1867. It was not
then published, as it was believed that the profession would not receive it favorably
until a sufficient number of living evidences in the shape of cures could be presented
as corroborative of its statements. That time has now come. It is highly gratify-
ing to find the following in the "Lancet," May 8, 1886, showing that other investigators are falling into line.

"PITYRIASIS AND PHTHISIS.

"Every physician is familiar with the cutaneous eruption occurring frequently on
the chest and back of phthisical patients, which passes under the name of pityriasis
versicolor, or chloasma, and the fact that it is due to the presence of a fungus allied
to those which cause favus and ringworm is well known ; but no one has at present sus-
pected that its presence had any significance, or that it had any real connection with
the essential lesion of phthisis. It was regarded as a fungus which took advantage,
so to speak, of the exhausted and debilitated condition of the patient, to take up its
abode in his skin, and it occurs in other wasting diseases of a similar nature. That
it is contagious, and can grow on the healthy skin is shown by the story which is
told of the French pathologist Lancereaux, who, wishing for the drawing of the
fungus for his plates on pathological anatomy, took some skin scrapings in an enve-
lope in his pocket, and was surprised after a time to find a plentiful crop of the par-
asite not only on his own chest but on that of his wife. But the fungus has now
come before us in a new light as playing a prominent part in the production of tubercular phthisis. According to the researches of M. M. Duguet and Héricourt,
the results of which were given to the Academy of Sciences on April 19, certain cases of acute tuberculosis presented no bacilli or zoogloea forms ; but when
the tissues were treated with potassium (ten to forty per cent.) a delicate mycelium

When the skin is filled with it, there ensues a loose soft state
of the skin with a disposition to constant perspiration, the sweat
smelling sour.   This keeps the surfaces of the body sticky and
subject to hot and cold flashes.   These spores, when in the skin,
have a bright nucleus, as seen in the illustration given further
on in Pl. XIV, Figs. 17, 18, 19, 20, 21, and 22.

The mycoderms develop largely throughout the digestive
organs.   In the second stage of the disease they pass from
these into the blood stream, where they multiply in masses
more or less oblong in shape.   When these masses get too large
to float through the pulmonary capillaries, they are caught
there and held fast, forming nuclei for subsequent tubercular
deposits.   After the mycoderms reach the blood stream, they
permeate every part and tissue of the body, marking the second stage of the disease.   From the fermenting foods in the
digestive organs they reach the mucous membranes of the air
passages, often before they pass to the blood stream.

From the beginning of the third stage, the whole organism

allied to that of microsporon was discovered ; and on pushing the inquiry further
it was found that this mycelium was more frequently present than the bacilli, being
seen not only in the tubercles but also in the neighboring healthy tissue. Similar
mycelial threads can also be found in the expectoration mixed with the bacilli.
When the microsporon furfur is cultivated and injected into guinea-pigs and rabbits,
these animals become without exception tuberculous, and the same result is obtained
by insufflation into the trachea of the crusts of pityriasis. Moreover, the cultures
of microsporon furfur, of tubercle produced from the fungus, and those from tubercles of man, are precisely the same in character. Cultivations can be made in
slightly alkalinized bouillon or in milk, when it becomes possible to distinguish an
ærobic and an anærobic element. The former floats at the surface, and at a temperature of from 30° to 38° C. forms a thick membrane composed of bacilli. The latter
is found at the bottom of the cultivation-tube as a mass of granulations and mycelium. The polymorphic character of the tubercle bacillus is thus manifest, and the
opinion of Spina receives support as to the variety of the forms of microcobes in
tuberculosis. The whole question is an interesting one, and it cannot be said to
be yet settled whether the various forms of low vegetable life to which we assign
names, are not phases in the life history of one species modified by chemical and physical conditions.

"The authors regard their discovery as important from the possibility of obtaining
an attenuated virus." — (*Lancet*, May 8, 1886.)

becomes more or less sour from the development of the myco-derms.

In the fourth or last stage this sour condition of the system is at its height.

The more exclusively the patient feeds upon fermenting foods, the more rapidly this vegetation develops in all parts of the body, and hastens the progress of the disease towards a fatal result.

X.

CONSUMPTION IS NOT AN INFLAMMATORY DISEASE.

CONSUMPTION, whether of the bowels, lungs or any other tissue or organ, is not an inflammatory disease, but is precisely the reverse, viz. : one of partial paralysis and interstitial starvation and death.

Whenever and wherever a mucous surface becomes partially paralyzed, from any injury or cause whatsoever, the follicles and surfaces begin at once to pour out a tough, ropy mucus which partially blocks up the follicles. Hence a stasis or congestion is produced in the enervated tissue, from the fact that this tough mucus does not flow freely out of the gland cells and tubes.

If continued for any great length of time this state of things produces hypernutrition of a low type of vitality and thickening of the parts. This we see in the catarrhal state of the membranes in the early stages of pulmonary phthisis and in the thick mucous secretions in the colon in consumption of the bowels (chronic diarrhœa).

If a man receives a blow on the back of the head near the base of the skull, so as to injure the pneumogastric nerve and to partially paralyze the branch going to the lungs, a thick, ropy mucus is immediately secreted from the pulmonary mucous membranes, and should he be so much paralyzed as to be unable to expectorate it, he soon fills up and suffocates. If, however, he is able to raise it, he may discharge from a pint to a quart or more in twenty-four hours, and this secretion keeps up until the paralysis disappears.

Now in consumption of the bowels or lungs the same paralyzed state exists. The paralysis in consumption, however, is not produced by a blow, but by the gradual presence and absorption from the stomach and bowels, of the mycoderma and the products developed by their growth and multiplication.

The most important factor in this paralysis is the absorption of carbonic acid gas, which is developed in the stomach in large quantities and is rapidly absorbed. In chronic diarrhœa, or consumption of the bowels, it is largely developed in the colon previous to and during the continuance of the diarrhœa.

It is this gas that is absorbed in the large bowel, which it so paralyzes that the bowel loses its normal peristaltic power to pass the fecal matters along, and they remain there fermenting, decaying and paralyzing till the organ becomes so filled with yeast, fermenting matters and jelly-like mucus — all in a state of active fermentation — that the bulky materials are forced out in numerous passages daily, the patient often having little or no power to retain them.

If the disease be permitted to continue for any great length of time, the colon becomes so thickened that the passage-way through it may not be one-fourth or even one-eighth of an inch in diameter, and in some cases it is entirely closed up. This thickening is not the result of inflammation, but of a partial paralysis of the parts, which results in a thick, ropy condition of the mucous secretions. This stringy gelatinous mucus is so thick that it cannot flow freely out of the follicles. In consequence the parts are dammed up and become more or less congested, under a state of partial death. This congested state results in hypernourishing, or overnourishing the parts, and excessive growth ensues.

The tissues (thickenings) organized under this condition have a low state of vitality and are liable to die and slough away under slight provocation.

XI.

THE STAGES IN CONSUMPTION.

First Stage.

THE FIRST, or incubative stage of consumption, is the fermentation of vegetable food, fruits, sweets and fats in the stomach and bowels, or in the feeding too freely and continuously upon the products of these various fermentations, by which the digestive apparatus becomes a veritable " yeast-pot," and all its follicles become filled with alcohol and the sour yeasts.

This state of things, if long continued, results in the partial paralysis of the cells of the follicles and villi of the digestive organs, so that the cells which take up food for nourishing the body lose little by little that normal selective power by virtue of which those products only are taken up that are required to support the tissues in a healthy manner. The impaired cells begin to " gobble " up carbonic acid gas, vinegar, vinegar yeast, and other deleterious bodies : this condition marks the beginning and gradual development of the *second stage* of consumption. In the first stage the blood becomes thinner, and more ropy and sticky, but is not much changed otherwise. During its progress there is a gradual increase of lassitude, with a tendency to tire and get out of breath, even in ordinary labors and exertions. There is a tendency to cold feet, to palpitation of the heart, dizzy head with, often, nervous, wakeful nights. This stage may continue from one to many years, depending upon the manner of living, the drinks, exercise, and other habits.

The first stage may be divided into three well-marked periods, which are tolerably well defined.

A. The first period of this stage is confined to fermentation of vegetables, breads, fruits and sweets in the stomach. This goes on for a longer or shorter time, according to the kind and character of the food and drinks, the exercise, exposure and habits. After this period has advanced sufficiently to paralyze the stomach and the valve [1] at the pyloric end of the organ, the fermenting food ceases to remain long in the stomach, on account of the relaxed and open condition of the pyloric valve which, up to this point, has been closed and unusually rigid. If the first period (*A*) of the disease continues for a long time, as it frequently does, during which time the stomach is constantly filled with carbonic acid gas (much of which may be eructated, but the greater part of which is absorbed), the heart, diaphragm, and portal organs become sluggish, enervated, and more or less paralyzed. The circulation grows weak ; the feet are cold, with a tendency to numbness ; head more or less dizzy and full ; portal glands and kidneys sluggish ; urine loaded with bile and lithates ; bowels often constipated ; breathing often oppressed ; pulse slow and often intermittent ; and in the later stages, the feet swell during the day. If this state of things be allowed to continue for any great length of time, there is great danger of fatty disease of the heart, and sometimes of fatty or amyloid disease of the liver and spleen. The cause of this fatty disease is the partial paralysis of these organs, which finally becomes so great that there is not sufficient vitality and action in the parts to bring to them their proper nourishment ; and nature, to prevent dissolution of the elements of the organs, infiltrates fat into them, by means of which they are preserved. Occasionally, in this period of the disease, the lobular or glycogenic portion of the liver becomes congested, by having the branch of

---

[1] When fermentation in the stomach first sets in, the pyloric valve closes with unusual force, so as to prevent the passage of the poisonous yeasts into the bowels below, and there is a tendency to eructate and throw up the fermenting products, till the whole organ becomes too much paralyzed to contract, when the pyloric valve relaxes and the fermenting materials pass readily into the small bowels, which ushers in the second stage of the disease.

the pneumogastric nerve, which goes to those parts, partially paralyzed ; this causes a stasis in the parts, which results in the formation of more animal sugar than the system requires. In this case the kidneys are called upon to eliminate it, and we have then the disease known as diabetes.

B. As soon as the pyloric valve ceases to retain the yeasty products in the stomach, they drop readily into the small bowels, which marks the second period of this first stage of the disease. In this period the patient experiences great relief in the stomach, (the acidity and gases not being retained in that organ) and expresses himself as being greatly improved. The fermentation is chiefly confined to the small bowels, during this period. After this has gone on for a longer or shorter time, according to circumstances, the ileo-cæcal valve becomes paralyzed, and the fermenting products readily pass into the colon, when chronic diarrhœa, or consumption of the bowels, sets in.

C. We have now entered upon the third period of the disease. This third period of the first stage of consumption may or may not occur.

Whether it occurs or not depends much upon the extent of the exclusive diet and drinks, and upon the habits of exercise, etc.

This third period of the first stage is represented in animals, in a marked degree, in the diarrhœa of the so-called " hog cholera," and in man in the " chronic diarrhœa " of armies, which in both cases are nothing more or less than " consumption of the bowels," or a well-established yeast pot in the colon. These discharges will ferment dough as well as will the sour yeast of the mash tub or the old yeast pot.

In the first, or incubative stage of consumption, where the diet, exercise, surrounding conditions and state of the system are such that the ileo-cæcal valve is not sufficiently paralyzed for a considerable period of time, (so as to allow the fermenting products to pass readily into the colon) the incubative stage remains in its second period, keeping the small bowels constantly filled with yeast. This soon paralyzes the cells of the villi to such an extent that they begin to take up the "sour yeasts," carbonic acid gas and other products of fermentation, all of which are transferred into the lacteal system and subsequently into the blood stream. Here the acid yeasts begin to aggregate and develop in masses or collects, which, as the spores multiply, increase in size to the diameter of the capillary vessels, when they begin to elongate, so that the masses often attain a length of from two to eight times their diameter. When they have attained a size sufficient to pass with difficulty through the capillary vessels of the lungs, they occasionally become fastened, fixed, and form the nuclei of future tubercles. It is when the incubative stage is arrested in its progress down the intestinal tract, and in its second period, that the dangers thicken, from the fact that this affords the yeast products an opportunity to get more readily into the blood stream, on account of their being blocked up in the small bowels.

When the sour yeasts have reached the blood stream, the spores gradually multiply and accumulate in little elongated masses, till they (the masses) get too large to pass through the pulmonary capillaries, when they begin to be caught up by them, and the lungs speedily become involved. Unless the causes are removed, the disease now advances to a fatal termination, usually within three years, while if the ileo-cæcal valve early becomes paralyzed, so as to let the yeast products drop readily and quickly into the colon, the danger of the yeast passing into the blood is greatly lessened, as it is then carried off daily in profuse diarrhœal discharges, and the patient may survive from one to twenty years with consumption of the bowels, before he is worn out, or before the lungs become seriously involved. The length of time that the patient lives depends upon his constitution, diet, exercise, habits and the surrounding conditions and circumstances.

Resumé of the First Stage of Consumption.

The first stage of consumption is confined exclusively to the digestive organs.

It consists in the alcoholic and acid fermentations of saccharine and farinaceous products, and in the fermentations of fats and glucose. These processes develop large amounts of carbonic acid gas (which gradually tends to paralyze the mucous surfaces) and also alcoholic, acetic, butyric, and other organic acids. Such products are the result of the development of vast multitudes of alcoholic, vinegar, butyric, acid and other yeast plants.

These plants belong to the genera Saccharomyces and Mycoderma.

The disease is confined to the bowels till the mucous surfaces become so paralyzed, under the influence of carbonic acid gas, (constantly present) that the cells lose their normal selective power, when the minute plants belonging to the genus Mycoderma begin to be " gobbled up " with the vinegar and carbonic acid gas, all of which now have a free and quite unobstructed pathway into the blood stream.

The passage of these products into the blood marks the beginning of the second stage of consumption.

XII.

THE SECOND STAGE, OR STAGE OF TRANSMISSION.

THIS is the stage of consumption when the yeast products are passing from the small intestines into the blood glands and the blood stream.

In the first stage the yeast (Mycoderma) products are confined to the stomach and bowels.

The first stage begins to lapse into the second as soon as the cells covering the villi become so paralyzed that they begin to lose that exquisite selective power by virtue of which those materials only are taken up from the alimentary canal which are needed for the support of the various tissues, and when the yeast products begin to enter the lacteals, lacteal glands and blood stream. Yeast now begins to accumulate in the blood glands and blood, and the whole system becomes unduly charged with carbonic acid gas, so that the heart, diaphragm, lungs and in fact the entire body, begin to become enervated (a step in the slow process of carbonic acid paralysis), so much so that all the processes requisite to the support of a healthy body are greatly deranged and interfered with.

This stage of the disease immediately precedes the fixing of those stationary deposits known as tubercle.

This second stage cannot be determined by the usual physical signs, but can readily be made out, or unmistakably indicated by careful microscopic examination of the blood. It may have a variable duration of from six months to one year, and may also extend itself over a period of from one to three and sometimes more years. Under ordinary circumstances it usually lasts about one year.

The earlier indications of this stage are a softened, sticky, stringy, pultaceous appearance of colored and colorless corpuscles, with shortening and increase in diameter of fibrin filaments, and with a softened state of the blood clots. The colorless corpuscles are less firm, seem to have less body and break down more readily than in health. The whole of the morphological elements of the blood begin to take on a more and more (so to speak) " rotten " condition.

The yeast spores (Mycoderma) are at first thinly scattered, and are either single or in tiny aggregations, too small to obstruct the capillary vessels, or to stop up the most minute follicles in the epithelial surfaces. As this stage advances, all the before-mentioned states and conditions become more and more marked, and the yeast masses (Mycoderma) are by degrees larger and more numerous, till the second stage is terminated by the blocking up of the capillary vessels and follicles with the enlarging yeast masses, thus ushering in the third stage of consumption, or the stage of tubercular depositions.

XIII.

THIRD STAGE, OR STAGE OF TUBERCULAR DEPOSITION.

TUBERCLE is a secondary product, and has its origin in accumulations of yeast spores in localities and under conditions where they cannot escape. In such case they form a heterologous deposit, around which, as a nucleus, other morphological elements and multiplying yeast spores accumulate. It is produced in the capillary vessels by aggregations, masses, collects or emboli of yeast spores (Mycoderma), which become so large as to block up these vessels, forming a nucleus around which accumulate sticky, colorless corpuscles, fibrin filaments and more yeast spores : in the follicles and air cells of the lungs it is induced by aggregations of yeast spores (Mycoderma) and mucous cells and filaments which become too large to escape: it is produced in the connective tissue by the accumulation of yeast spores (Mycoderma) and connective tissue cells and fibres.

All these deposits continue to grow by accretions so long as vitality subsists in the morphological elements of the tubercle and its surroundings. When this vitality becomes extinct, the tubercle gradually softens and finally breaks down, or — if the process is very slow and slight vitality still inheres in it and in the surrounding parts — it undergoes fatty infiltration, which preserves it from readily breaking down.

This third stage continues through a period varying in length with the diet, surroundings, exercise, constitution and constitutional diathesis of the patient. Its limits in duration are from one to three years. The average would fall short of two years.

This period is terminated by the gradual ushering in of the fourth stage, or period of interstitial death, decay and disintegration, which is the final stage of the disease.

XIV.

FOURTH STAGE, OR STAGE OF INTERSTITIAL DEATH, SOFTENING,
DECAY AND DISINTEGRATION.

THE fourth stage of consumption may be preceded by fatty infiltration and fatty metamorphosis, and, in cases of "gravel of the lungs," — or in a gravelly diathesis, — fatty infiltration and fatty metamorphosis may be followed, and the breaking-down stage preceded by the period of calcification.

The fourth stage is a well-defined one, and is always indicated by variable, chilly feelings during the early part of the day, followed by more or less fever in the middle and after-part, and by cold, more or less profuse sweating at night.

The severity of the algid, hot and sweating conditions is indicative of the rapidity of the interstitial death, decay and breaking down of lung tissue.

During this stage the patient is dying faster than he is living. Decay is making greater inroads than his materials suffice to repair.

If at any time the digestion and assimilation so far improve that blood is made faster than it is used up, lung repair goes on more rapidly than does the breaking-down process, and the chills, fever and sweats, growing lighter by degrees, soon cease entirely. When this repair takes place faster than the disintegration, the curative process is in progress, and if it keeps on, and accidents are avoided, the patient will get well. His cure is then merely a question of time and of continuance in right doing, with soul and body, in carrying on the good work.

This stage is ushered in by the gradual interstitial death and

disintegration of cells and fibres of the lung tissue, which disintegrated cells and connective tissue fibres are expectorated,
and may be found more or less abundantly in all the sputa.

This gradual breaking down and death indicates a low state
of vitality, and is accompanied by great lassitude and weakness,
with chills, fevers and sweats as before stated. These are outward manifestations of this slow death and decay. The blood
is not being made as fast as it is being used up, and a slow,
steady, progressive starvation process sets in. Unless this process can be checked by such feeding as will improve digestion
and assimilation, and make sufficient blood to repair waste more
rapidly than the breaking down tissues can cause waste, this
stage of the disease will certainly and quickly end in death.

We are thus led to the only true and sure method of curing
consumption, which is by removing its cause — (fermenting
food) — and putting the patient on a rigid unfermentative diet,
coupled with such a process of outside and inside cleansing, as
will get the " machine clean," sweet and in good running order.

XV.

IMPOSSIBLE TO DETERMINE THE PRESENCE OF CONSUMPTION
BY AUSCULTATION AND PERCUSSION, IN THE FIRST TWO
STAGES OF THE DISEASE.

IN the incubative and transmissive stages of consumption, it is seldom that auscultation and percussion afford any clue to the condition of the patient. These means are only of service in throwing light upon the state of the lungs after deposits have begun to take place.

Before any deposits occur, there may be a period of considerable duration, when no outward physical signs of the disease present themselves, except that the patient becomes readily fatigued; the pulse abnormally slow, normal in frequency or rapid, but in all cases weak; the breathing is accelerated, the patient complaining that he cannot breathe deeply enough, and hence taking frequently a long breath; weak and often painful sensations in the region of the heart and left shoulder - blade; oppression about the chest, with a secretion of tough, ropy mucus in throat and bronchial tubes; a marked tendency to take cold on the least exposure, with cold feet and hands. There is also an impaired power of lung expansion from weakened respiratory action, caused by partial paralysis of the pulmonary tissues, diaphragm and other respiratory muscles, which paralysis is brought about by absorption of the fermenting products from stomach and bowels. The microscope is our unerring guide during these two prior stages of the disease, which, taken together, represent the pretubercular stage. The microscopic appearance of the blood indicates with precision the condition of the patient, and the progress he has made in the disease.

XVI.

CONSUMPTION OF THE BOWELS, OR CHRONIC DIARRHŒA.

THIS disease, with the other intercurrent abnormal states that arise from a too exclusive use of an amylaceous and saccharine diet, etc., may be conveniently divided into three stages; viz.: The Incubative, Acute and Chronic.

1. *The Incubative Stage.*

In all cases uncomplicated by dysentery, intermittent and remittent fevers, etc., the diarrhœa is preceded by a constipated condition of the bowels. This, however, is overlooked by the patient, from the fact that in many cases the diarrhœa comes on gradually: there is at first but one profuse passage in twenty-four hours, and this takes place in the latter part of the night, or early in the morning.

The appetite being good, and there being no pains, — save immediately preceding the passage, — this condition is frequently allowed to run on for some time uncared for, and till the passages have increased from four to ten or more per day, taking place mostly during the latter part of the night and morning hours. The patient now applies for treatment and almost invariably reports that his diarrhœa has been preceded by looseness.

The incubative stage of the disease has made no impression upon him, and he only remembers that his bowels have been loose for some time. If his case be carefully traced back however, a preliminary constipated period will be found to have existed. This period has often been of several weeks' standing. During this constipation the patient has had from one to four scant, difficult and either hard or plastic passages per week. During the evening and night he has been troubled with the development of gases in his stomach and bowels, often distending these organs so as to excite pain through from one side to the other, accompanied by eructations and passages of wind.

Often the bowels and stomach become so paralyzed that the patient is unable to eructate or pass the generating gases, and hence he frequently becomes enormously distended.

This development of gases in the alimentary canal goes on increasing during the incubative stage till diarrhœa sets in. During this constipated condition there is also a paralytic tendency.

This first shows itself in the large intestines, in a want of normal sensibility and peristaltic action, and then in the lower extremities, which exhibit prickling sensations and are liable to "get asleep," as the patients describe it. There is a mixed up, numb feeling in the head, often with a confused condition; ringing in the ears at night and muscæ volitantes, with sometimes a blur before the eyes and defective or dulled memory.

The bronchial and pulmonary membranes display more or less irritation, frequently attended with a feeling of constriction about the chest, with a cough during the night and towards morning, and often with expectoration of thick, cream-colored, sweetish mucus after rising. The tongue is in general unusually clean and watery, with a red border and a red streak down the centre, which central streak sometimes feels sore. There is often palpitation of the heart on slight exertions, with a tendency to fibrinous depositions in the heart and the large vessels leading to it. The voice becomes often hoarse and husky, with a peculiar, stiff, constricted feeling in the pharyngeal and laryngeal region. There is a lassitude about the muscles which is rather dispelled than otherwise on taking exercise. Appetite good and often ravenous for fermenting foods.

With many persons the symptoms of the incubative stage are not very strongly marked, especially when such patients are actively engaged. After a short time, in such cases, it frequently passes away, the alimentary canal adapting itself to the dry amylaceous and saccharine food, so that digestion goes on quite passably to all appearances, and the passages become quite natural in consistence, color and frequency. When this period is once passed, the tendency to have diarrhœa from living upon beans, crackers and other fermentable foods is much lessened, and the patients are now disposed to become more plethoric than usual. They feel, however, less tonicity of the system and readily tire; they are frequently troubled with palpitations, and short, hurried and often oppressed breathing after any severe fatigue. If, however, the system becomes debilitated through any cause, such as typhoid, intermittent and remittent fevers, etc., there is a marked tendency to diarrhœic conditions, which, if not early subdued, becomes chronic and more difficult to control. There is in such cases a marked tendency for the lungs to become involved in the disease, whenever — from any cause — the digestion and assimilation are impaired.

Quite frequently cases are met with of remarkably strong and vigorous digestive organs, where the paralytic tendencies of the incubative stage continue without exciting diarrhœa. In such cases there is a marked tendency to fibrinous depositions in and near the heart, (thrombosis,) and to the gradual tearing loose of these thrombi and their lodgment as emboli in the pulmonary capillaries, producing congestions and smothering sensations. There is also a tendency to tubercular depositions and paralytic diseases of the eye and ear, with partial paralysis of the larynx and pains and aches of a neuralgic character in the extremities and back. Such patients are soon disabled and become permanent invalids, and not many months elapse before the abnormal states advance so far that the diseased conditions become obstinate and difficult to cure. Frequently this class of patients become so paralyzed that they are unable to help themselves. In others, aching symptoms present themselves in all parts of the body ; these are neuralgic in character, and indicate an ener-

vated and paralytic tendency. This is due to the long continued development in the digestive organs of yeast vegetations
and carbonic acid gas, which being absorbed, have partially
paralyzed the entire nervous system.

2. *Acute Stage.*

The incubative stage is followed by a looseness of the bowels
or a diarrhœa more or less marked, with large development of
gaseous products in the stomach and intestines, particularly
during the evening and night.

The first diarrhœa generally comes on towards morning.
Usually there is at first but a single passage daily, and this
occurs in the latter part of the night or early in the morning.
Much wind is passed with it. Before the passage and immediately after, there is a heat and throbbing in the lower portion
of the large intestines. The evacuation is followed by a general feeling of relief and usually there is no uneasiness about
the bowels during the subsequent day. Nothing abnormal is
felt till the following evening, when the stomach and intestines
become again distended with flatus, which appears in active
motion. This continues through the night or until the profuse
evacuation, which is generally more watery than that of the
first night, and is accompanied and followed by the same train
of symptoms.

This state of things may continue, with but slight increase,
for from two to ten days, according to the food, exercise and
condition of the system. Finally, the bloating during the night
and the passages following and accompanying the same become
so frequent and disturb the rest of the patient so much that he
applies for medical treatment. During the acute stage there is
a highly fermentative tendency in the alimentary canal during
the evening and night, accompanied by more or less pain. The
passages at this period frequently and suddenly increase from
one or two daily, to twenty or more. In a few hours the patient becomes reduced so low that he is unable to get up alone,

and the large intestines and sphincter become so paralyzed that the feces are passed involuntarily in bed. This is particularly the case in armies. All of these conditions are, however, met with almost daily in private practice. This is especially the case in zymotic regions, or localities where cryptogamic vegetations and fermentations readily occur and progress rapidly.

The paralytic tendency, the ringing in the ears and the pulmonary and bronchial symptoms are more marked in the second than in the incubative or first stage. The heart becomes irritable, and is often thrown into violent palpitation by excitement. The tongue becomes red, swollen and smooth, or loose and watery. The voice is often husky and sometimes reduced to a whisper. Neuralgic pains occur in the extremities and back, and the urine becomes scanty and often loaded with oxalate of lime and cystine.

During this stage, which lasts for several days (the time varying with the diet, exercise and condition of the patient), the disease yields readily, as a general thing, to a simple cathartic dose of Rochelle salts, followed by the vegetable acid salts of potassa, soda and iron in dilute solutions, and a rigid diet of broiled lean beef, with one cup of clear tea at each meal. If neglected however, or if attempts are made to suppress it with opium and astringents, and with light farinaceous diet, the abnormal alimentary conditions invariably become worse, and the diarrhœa reappears with aggravated symptoms, and soon becomes chronic. There is more or less paralysis and congestion of a low type of the whole alimentary canal, and especially of the stomach and large intestines, which gradually take on a catarrhal condition, and become more or less thickened.

The discharges are thin and foamy, like yeast, filling a large chamber, very much to the surprise of both patient and attendant. These passages, however, weigh but little. In color they are either clayey, brownish, pinkish or normal, and contain more or less mucous and gelatinous (colloid) matter: the latter is disseminated through the fecal matters in little jelly-like lumps. Blood is frequently present in the later stages. Fragments of undigested food and crystals of triple phosphates, oxalate of lime and cystine are scattered abundantly through the stools.

Fragments of intestinal epithelium and casts (Plate I, Figs. 1, 2 and 3) of the follicles of the large bowels are found abundantly in the jelly-like mucus which is poured out from the follicles of these parts.

3. *Chronic Stage.*

During the chronic stage the stools range from three to twenty, or sometimes more, per day.

They occur more frequently during the night and morning than during the balance of the day, and are preceded and accompanied by the development, eructation and passage of much flatus.

Frequently the intestines are so thoroughly paralyzed that the patients are unable to pass or eructate the carbonic acid gas, it remaining and distending the abdomen to a most uncomfortable extent, and is gradually more or less absorbed. The intestinal gases are, as a rule, constantly in motion up and down, and are as constantly being developed.

During the day the passages are less frequent, especially during the latter half, and pending this time there is less flatus and uneasiness. The appetite is generally good — sometimes unusually so — there being no difficulty in retaining food on the stomach. Often the patients are hungry most of the time, and in some instances they desire to eat constantly, the food running through them almost as fast as taken, fermenting but undigested. Really the patients are starving to death, the alimentary canal being more a yeast pot than an apparatus for digesting food.

The passages are either chiefly of a pale yellow or ash color, and sometimes brownish green ; they are thin and watery, foamy and mushy or gelatinous and slimy. Lumps of gelatinous (colloid) matter, frequently streaked with blood, and sometimes masses of cream-colored pus, are disseminated through the stools in greater or lesser abundance, according to the severity of the case. The jelly-like mucus is more or less filled with algæ, closely allied to plants belonging to the genera Microcystis and Sirocoleum. These are probably present more as the consequence of certain conditions, than as causes of them. They are represented in Plate I, Figs. 26, 27, 28, 29 and 30; also in Plate II, Figs. 17 and 18.

The pus in the feces is distinguished from the slimy mucus by being thin and creamy, readily diffusing itself through water. The gelatinous mucus, or colloid matter, is glairy and ropy, like the white of an egg, and does not mix with water. It has either a clear, yellowish, greenish or brownish tinge, and occurs in lumps and ropes disseminated through the fecal matters when these have a sufficient consistence; and is readily distinguished from the ordinary mucus which covers the outside of consistent feces with a slimy layer. When the feces have not such consistence, the colloid matter is so mixed with them as scarcely to be distinguished, save by the ropiness and slimy character of the passages.

Other symptoms during this stage are as follows : —

Epigastrium. — More or less uneasiness, pain and swelling ; tenderness.

Colon and Rectum. — Constant tenderness, especially during the night.

Intestines and Sphincter. — In severe cases there is often complete paralysis of these, so that the feces are passed involuntarily in bed. Frequently in such cases the passages are almost entirely composed of gelatinous matter, which is sometimes of a dark, dirty hue, green by reflected light, and a greenish yellow by transmitted light. This matter is often mistaken for bilious secretion. The paralytic tendency observable during this stage shows itself more or less in the lower bowels, inferior extremities and head.

Heart. — Irregular and interrupted heart beat. Increased disposition to functional and organic disease of this organ, with strongly marked symptoms.

Lungs. — There is more or less bronchial and pulmonary irritation, with morning cough and expectoration of a sweetish, cream-colored mucus. An oppressed, constricted feeling in one or both lungs, and a marked tendency to the clogging up of pulmonary vessels with emboli and tubercular depositions.

Appetite. — Variable, though remarkably good in general, considering the gravity of the lesions. There is often an increased craving for food and drinks, but the food, notwithstanding the amount consumed, produces no increase of flesh. On the contrary, a steadily increasing emaciation is almost always noticed, with gradual enervation of body and mind.

Mouth, etc. — There is considerable thirst, a watery state of the mouth and fauces, or sometimes a greater dryness. Tongue unusually clean as a rule; often red and watery and sometimes bloody. The gums sometimes assume a reddish, spongy appearance and bleed readily. The breath is very offensive. There is often a peculiar constricting sensation in the pharynx in going through the act of swallowing.

Urine. — Small; sometimes loaded with lithates and oxalates.

Feces. — Offensive, fermentative odor.

Skin. — Dry, harsh, bran-like and scaly.

General Symptoms. — The general temperature of the body is lowered. Frequent chilliness is intermitted by occasional flashes of heat. There is a general sense of weariness; a "goneness" and sinking feeling, and great indisposition to bodily or mental exertion. The legs are very apt to prickle and "fall asleep," as the patient terms it. Ringing in the ears is frequent at night, and there is also an amaurotic tendency, with ulceration of the cornea, especially in advanced states of the disease. Dull pain and heat about the lower bowels; more or less pain and weakness in the lower extremities and back. If the disease be not checked, a daily increasing emaciation sets in. The patients become peevish, fretful, complaining and hypochondriacal, magnifying their pains and sensations. Palpitation of the heart, with oppressed breathing on lying down, become troublesome symptoms. There is often irritation, to a greater or lesser extent, in the bladder and urethra, with icteroid tendencies. The memory often becomes impaired and the patients more or less childish. There is a disagreeable exhalation from the surface of the body and from the pulmonary membranes.

Dyspeptic Symptoms.—These show themselves, especially during the evening and night, in acidity of the stomach ; sour eructations ; distention of the stomach and intestines with flatus, which is in constant motion in all directions, — a continual boiling and bubbling ; oppression and weight in the epigastrium ; burning sensations about the pericardia, etc.

In this stage of the complaint there is a remarkable tendency to tubercular depositions in the lungs, with the usual attendant symptoms. The patient sinks rapidly, the emaciation and debility become extreme, and sometimes what appears to be a peculiar diphtheritic exudation — but which is really alcoholic yeast plants (Saccharomyces) developing in the glycogenic mucous secretions — shows itself creeping up in the pharynx and fauces, and finally dips down into the larynx, and the patient soon expires, apparently exhausted from want of nourishment, which, although taken freely, is not appropriated, and passes in the feces mostly undigested.

Often, sometime before death, the entire epithelial surfaces of the body are found full of the spores of the Saccharomyces, which occasionally result in scabby sores.

XVII.

MICROSCOPIC EXAMINATION OF FECES IN CONSUMPTION OF THE BOWELS.

MICROSCOPIC and chemical examinations connected with the fecal discharges, developed the following conclusions : —

1. That after beginning to subsist on amylaceous and saccharine diet, and as soon as gases begin to develop in the stomach and bowels, the development of yeast plants is indicated in the alimentary canal matters to an abnormal extent.

2. That this development of yeast plants (Saccharomyces and Mycoderma) is evidence of the inauguration of fermentative changes in the amylaceous and saccharine foods.

3. That the development of the yeast plants belonging to the genera Saccharomyces and Mycoderma goes on increasing until diarrhœic conditions are produced.

4. That a peculiar, gelatinous, colloid matter — usually found in little masses scattered through the feces — shows itself to a greater or lesser extent as soon as the diarrhœa commences. That generally this matter is present in direct proportion to the severity of the case.

5. That this colloid matter, or jelly-like mucus, is not the cause of the diarrhœa, but is merely the consequence of continuous fermentation of amylaceous and saccharine foods in the large bowels, which causes the mucous membrane and connective tissue layers of this organ to thicken from the partial paralysis of the parts. The partial paralysis, the thickening and the catarrhal state of the parts, are all caused by the development of yeast plants and the consequent products. As soon as patients are put upon an exclusive diet of the pulp of lean beef, the yeast plants are killed or cleaned out, the fermenta-

tive changes cease, and the thickened state together with the attendant catarrhal condition gradually pass away, and a healthy state is restored.

6. That the system generally becomes charged with fermenting saccharine, alcoholic and acid matters, so that these products may be found in all the mucous and skin secretions, together with the vegetations (Mycoderma and Saccharomyces) developing in them. In all three stages of the disease, sugar, alcohol, and acetic, butyric and lactic acids are found largely present in the fecal discharges.

Sugar in Fecal Matter and in Mucous Secretions.

In all three stages of consumption of the bowels, sugar is largely present in the fecal matters and in the mucous secretions of the alimentary canal.

Fatty products, and crystals of the triple phosphates and oxalate of lime are also frequently present in· the stools in large quantities.

Alcoholic yeast is abundant, and frequently the developing spores of a species of penicilium : sometimes also the cells of the sarcina ventriculi are met with.

All these are indications of active fermentative changes in the saccharine and amylaceous matters present. The large development of gaseous products during the evening and night, is indicative of active fermentation of amylaceous food eaten during the day.

There is evidence that the secretions of the mucous membrane of the alimentary canal, fauces, mouth and pulmonary surfaces, eventually become saccharine. This is shown in the development of saccharomyces and filaments of penicilium in the viscid layer of mucus lining the whole alimentary canal, and in the mucous secretions of the œsophagus, pharynx, larynx, tracheæ and mouth in the later stages of the disease. This development on the surface of the fauces, pharynx and mouth resembles the exudation in diphtheria, for which it is frequently taken.

Beautiful hexagonal prisms of crystalline sugar are frequently met with in the fecal matters.

Cholesterin and Serolin in Feces.

Cholesterin and serolin occur quite largely in the feces of chronic diarrhœa, the latter in greater quantity than the former. The longer the feces stand and ferment — whether in or out of the bowels — the less cholesterin there is and the more serolin.

Cryptogamic Vegetation in Feces.

The spores of the yeast plant (Saccharomyces, Pl. I, Figs. 31 and 33 ; Pl. II, Fig. 35) occur largely in the fecal matters of every well-marked case of chronic diarrhœa. There are also the cells of what appears to be a larger species of Saccharomyces. These are not uniformly met with.

The sarcina ventriculi or " wool sack " plant is often found present in large quantities.

Such cases are the more obstinate ones, there being greater difficulty in checking the abnormal development of intestinal gases.

There is also another species of sarcina which I have occasionally met with. The cells are smaller and more pearly than those of the ventriculi, and usually occur singly, or in twos, and sometimes in fours. (Pl. I, Fig. 34.)

Two or three species of minute algæ occur abundantly in all well-marked cases. (Pl. II, Figs. 12, 38, 40 and 41.)

Occasionally the vegetating spores and mycelium of a species of penicilium (Pl. II, Figs. 20 and 23) are met with in the colloid matter, especially in cases where the stools are mainly made up of this gelatinous substance and are of a greenish color.

This colloid or gelatinous matter is uniformly present in all true cases of chronic diarrhœa. It occurs, however, in much larger quantities in the stools of persons living in malarious localities than in those of persons resident in non-malarious districts.

XVIII.

POST-MORTEM APPEARANCES, STATES AND CONDITIONS, IN CON-
SUMPTION OF THE BOWELS OR CHRONIC DIARRHŒA, IN THE
HUMAN SUBJECT.

Lungs. — These are usually more or less invaded by either
the clogging of the pulmonary vessels with small fibrinous clots
(emboli), or tubercular deposits in the lung tissue, or both.

When the disease has continued for a great length of time,
scarcely an instance is found where there is an entire absence of
lung complication. The pulmonary and bronchial membranes
present indications of more or less irritation, and frequently
something like an exudation is noticed creeping up the pharynx
into the fauces, and then dipping down into the larynx and
tracheæ. This apparent exudation is not one in fact, it being
composed — in every case I have met with — of alcoholic and
organic acid yeast plants, held together by filamentous mucus,
all of which indicate a saccharine or glycogenic and fermentative condition of the mucous membranes and their secretions.
These apparent exudations, composed of yeast plants, creep up,
as I have said, along the œsophagus into the pharynx and
fauces, and then dip down into the larynx and tracheæ. They
are unfavorable indications and appear in the most marked degree a few days previous to death. They are more prominent
in cases of chronic diarrhœa which have accompanied and followed typhoid fever.

The fecal matter of such patients is invariably filled with
large globules of fat, many of which are covered with a crystalline crust, from which radiate acicular crystals in all directions. These acicular crystals resemble ciliæ, giving to the

large fat globules the appearance of being ciliated bodies. (Pl. II, Figs. 19 and 19¹.) The lungs are frequently found filled with small tubercles and sometimes large ones, in process of disintegration. At other times the lungs may either contain tubercles or not, and are more or less hepatized, the congestion being a direct result of emboli which have lodged in the minute pulmonary vessels, damming up the blood and preventing its free passage.

Heart. — The heart is nearly, if not always more or less involved in the disease. There is a disposition to fibrinous deposits in the cavities of the heart and the vessels leading to and therefrom, producing the disease described by Virchow as thrombosis.

Granules, layers, conical masses and ropes of fibrin — usually of a white color — are found attached to the internal surface of the cavities of the heart around the valves, also ropes of fibrin sometimes extend out into the vessels leading therefrom. There is often more or less effusion into the pericardium as well.

Kidneys. — The kidneys, as a general rule, present no marked organic lesions. They are, however, almost constantly deranged in functions, which sometimes results in organic disease.

Œsophagus. — The œsophagus is often congested and apparently inflamed. It is frequently covered with mucus filled with yeast cells and spores of a species of penicilium vegetation, forming a coating to the mucous surface which is not unlike a diphtheritic exudation.

Stomach. — The walls of the stomach are usually thickened ; the tubular glands are more or less enlarged, and they are sometimes found projecting beyond the walls in small fungoid-looking masses, wider above and constricted below. These little elevations are from one to several lines in diameter, and rise from one quarter to half a line above the surface. They frequently run together, forming larger or smaller patches, and sometimes are thickly set over the entire internal surface of the stomach, appearing not very unlike exudations, except that they have a reddish, vascular appearance. In cleaning the stomach they are liable to be brushed or torn off, leaving ragged or clean edged depressions, resembling the bed of ulcers. In this way many stomachs which have been examined only after cleaning, seem to have been ulcerated, when really no such lesions existed. The final tendency of the follicular enlargements is to disintegrate, leaving ulcers. Ulceration, however, takes place in comparatively few cases, even where the diarrhœa causes death.

These follicular enlargements are the outcome of a partially paralyzed state of the follicles, from the constant presence of carbonic acid gas and other yeast products. As soon as a mucous membrane becomes partially paralyzed, a thick, ropy mucus begins to be secreted and poured out. When this is so thick and abundant as to clog the follicles, a stasis in the parts is the result, and under a low state of vitality the connective and mucous tissues begin to thicken.

This thick, gelatinous mucus not only resembles, but is actually closely allied in cause, composition, genesis and development to the colloid matter of goitre and ovarian disease.

The intervening spaces on the mucous lining of the stomach, not occupied by the enlarged follicles, are usually more or less of a red-beefy, ash or slate color, and sometimes greenish, indicating what appears to be either a stasis or high stage of congestion of a low type of vitality, — or anæmic, deadened condition. The walls of the stomach are generally covered with an adherent, slimy, greasy layer, which appears to prevent the food from coming in direct contact with its mucous surface. The internal gastric walls are usually more or less thickened and red. The organ is frequently diminished in size, sometimes to one-third or one-fourth its normal capacity.

Small Intestines. — The mucous lining of the small intestines is usually covered with a thin, slimy, adherent layer of fecal matter, mucous and oily products, which stick so closely that they are only removed by washing and scraping. This is a layer of alcoholic yeasts and decaying food, and is very offensive. With the exception of this layer, these intestines are entirely empty of fecal matter, but are distended with fetid gases. On the removal of this offensive coating, the mucous membrane is generally quite normal in appearance, save that here and there are congested streaks and patches. The ulcerations, when they occur, are chiefly in the lower part of the ilium, near the cœcal valve.

Large Intestine. — This is usually very much thickened, and the internal surface is covered with a thin, dirty yellow, pultaceous layer of slimy, fecal matter, very offensive in odor and feeling greasy to the touch. This adheres so closely to the intestinal walls that it is removed only by washing and scraping. It is filled with alcoholic and acid yeast vegetations, and frequently with the spores of a species of penicilium, with gelatinous matter; sometimes also with the sarcina ventriculi: (Pl. I, Fig. 34.) These were found to be more numerous towards the stomach than lower down.

The inner wall of the large intestine along its whole length, and that of about one inch of the lower part of the ilium adjacent to the cœcal valve, are generally found to be more or less thickly studded with ragged patches or fungoid elevations, from one to two lines in diameter and elevated above the surface from about one-fourth to one-half line. These patches are wide above and constricted below, and are composed of the enlarged intestinal follicles and gelatinous matters. In many instances two or more of these patches are found united, forming larger elevations. In cleaning the intestines many of these fungoid elevations are torn off, producing ragged-edged depressions not unlike the bed of ulcers. These enlarged, highly congested and vascular follicles are connected with the formation of colloid matter. This matter is more or less tinged with yellow and green. It is found disseminated in small lumps and ropes through the feces. In some of the worst forms of the disease, the passages are composed almost entirely of this colloid matter. In such cases it is usually of a dirty green color by reflected light, and a dirty, greenish-yellow by transmitted light. The solitary glands are enlarged, and are the seat of a bluish-black pigment, which readily points out their location. Frequently these fungoid elevations disintegrate, leaving ulcers in their places. Such ulcers are met with of a large size in many fatal cases. Ulceration, however, is not as frequent in this disease as is generally supposed. The inner walls of the intestine frequently become largely thickened, and the calibre lessened. The intervals not occupied by the fungoid elevations are highly congested and apparently inflamed, having a peculiar dark, beef-red color. Sometimes cases occur where the mucous lining of the large intestines is merely of a beef-red color, without any fungoid elevations. In others, the beef-red patches are found mingled with patches that are greenish, slate-colored or brownish. The intestinal capillaries are more or less clogged up with emboli, which prevent the free passage of blood, and from which results the peculiar congestion and consequent thickening, the absorbent power of the intestinal walls being more or less impaired or destroyed.

Mesenteric Glands. — The mesenteric glands of the small intestines are always enlarged, congested, softened and gorged with blood in proportion to the intestinal lesion.

Omentum. — The omentum is in general entirely deprived of adipose, and is red and highly congested.

Spleen. — The spleen is always more or less enlarged, filled with liquid blood and softened.

Liver. — The liver, as a general rule, is quite healthy and firm. It has more of a yellowish tinge than is normal, but it is otherwise usually natural in appearance, except when a diabetic condition supervenes, in which case the lobules are more or less congested.

Pathology of the Disease.

This, as indicated by :

A. The microscopic examinations of fecal matters ; *B.* Of the lining membrane and capillaries of the alimentary canal ; *C.* Of the pulmonary and cerebral capillary vessels ; and *D.* Of the heart ; consists :

1. In the development of fermentative changes in the amylaceous food retained an undue time in the alimentary canal, by which yeast plants, carbonic acid and the other products of fermentation are largely developed.

2. The fermentative changes and the continued feeding upon an amylaceous food, eventually result in a highly saccharine or glycogenic and fermentative condition of the system. This fermentative condition tends at first to accelerate cell development and cell transformation.

3. In the spleen, mesenteric glands and blood-vessels, the fibrin cells are more rapidly developed and transformed into tough sticky fibrin, which has a strong tendency to become organized and aggregated into masses. Hence fibrinous deposits result in the heart, producing the thrombosis of Virchow, and numerous clots (emboli) form and become fixed in the capillary blood-vessels of such parts as are the most sensitive and irritable, and the most irritated. These clots increase and soon obstruct the free passage of the blood through such irritated parts, damming them up, producing congestions in the intestinal walls, mesenteric glands and spleen, with more or less congestion and hepatization of the lungs from the accumulation of emboli in the pulmonary capillaries.

4. From the tendency to cell multiplication, produced by the fermentative state of the system, there is a marked disposition to the development of tubercles in the lungs.

5. The disease is, primarily, eminently a fermentative one, tending to produce blood clots in the heart and capillary vessels, from which result a variety of peculiar, almost painless congestions and chronic inflammations, with paralytic conditions.

6. The clogging up of the intestinal capillaries destroys to a greater or lesser extent the normal power of the intestinal walls; hence the impossibility for the alimentary membranes to either pour out the materials that aid in forming chyme and in producing healthy digestion, or to take up nutrient products. In these cases the conditions are such as to tend to imperfect nutrition and finally to starvation.

7. From the clogging up of the intestinal capillaries with emboli (fibrinous clots), the follicles and villi become highly congested, and a chronic enlargement of these organs soon ensues. As they enlarge they protrude — often in patches — beyond the level of the mucous surface, frequently forming fungoid elevations, wider above and constricted below. These somewhat resemble patches of exudation, and with the surrounding and subjacent connective tissue, take on a peculiar abnormal action resembling that of some forms of tumors where a gelatinous (colloid) matter is developed. There are two forms of the colloid or gelatinous disease occurring in the human body; one as a tumor, the other as an infiltration. The latter is more common in the alimentary canal, particularly in the stomach and large intestines. It also occurs sometimes in the bladder. The former (tumor) occurs in the glandular organs, peritoneum, omentum, cellular tissue, thyroid gland, ovary and bones. In the infiltrated variety, the gelatinous matter occupies the meshes of the cellular substance, forming cysts from the size of a mustard seed to that of a hazelnut, which are filled with characteristic jelly-like matter, and which as they increase in volume, so completely subvert the primitive substance as ultimately to leave no trace of it. This colloid or gelatinous matter is either colorless, whitish, yellowish or greenish, and has usually the consistence of jelly.

It emanates from partially paralyzed epithelial and connective tissue elements. Virchow rather objects to the term *colloid*, preferring the term *mucus*. The matter does not, however, resemble mucus nearly so much as it does gelatine, to which it bears a close resemblance in appearance. When the so-called colloid matter is developed in connective tissue, the growth (which appears to be allied to homœoplasia) is not usually of that malignant type which it assumes when it is (heteroplasia) developed in bone, cartilage or other tissue not yielding gelatine normally.

8. These colloid growths, when seated on mucous surfaces, appear in the enlarged form of follicles, villi, papillæ or warts. These are precisely the forms presented in chronic diarrhœa, studding the surface of the large intestines, and often of the stomach; frequently also the lower portion of the ilium. They give rise to or develop large quantities of colloid matter, which is formed abundantly, and scattered through the fecal discharges in lumps and ropes. In the later stages of severe cases, sometimes almost the entire evacuations are made up of this matter, which is either nearly transparent, or else of a dark, dirty-green color by reflected light, and of a dirty, greenish-yellow hue by transmitted light.

In bronchocele a similar colloid matter is developed. The same substance is also formed in a peculiar, quite fatal form of chronic vesico-renal inflammation. In this disease the bladder is found to be studded with the same kind of fungoid elevations as exist in the large intestines of chronic diarrhœa. Frequently in chronic diarrhœa these fungoid elevations disintegrate, leaving in their places ulcerated depressions, in which cases pus — frequently streaked with blood — will be found in the feces. Ulceration, as before stated, is not so frequent, however, as is generally supposed. In cleaning the intestines for wet preparations, the fungoid elevations are often torn off, leaving either smooth or ragged-edged depressions resembling ulcers. These are often taken for points of ulceration.

9. The diseased portions of the alimentary lining are a dark, livid red, a slate color, ash color or greenish shade. The solitary follicles are enlarged, and are frequently the seat of pigment deposits, so that the locality of each can be readily recog-

nized by the unaided eye from the presence of a bluish-black dot.

Every and all remedial means that have a tendency to produce an astringent, soporific or congestive influence, aggravate the disease.

The great and primary objects are to subdue the fermentative tendency; to dissolve the aggregated masses of fibrin in the clogged-up capillaries, and to supply that kind of diet, the want of which has caused the disease. Hence the reason why an albuminous animal diet, with non-amylaceous, anti-fermentative vegetables in small quantity and the vegetable acid salts of the alkalies and iron, are so valuable and produce such charmed results.

Cause. — The primary cause of the so-called chronic diarrhœa appears to be vegetable and especially amylaceous diet. In armies this diet consists of dry bread or biscuit, with sweetened coffee or tea. Upon a careful and extensive examination, it has been found that when soldiers are on the march, they are obliged to live mainly upon the army biscuit, from the fact that they can only carry cooked meats for a few days' rations and cannot usually carry the means for cooking on the way. The result is that the dry biscuit constitutes their main food for a considerable portion of the time. This dry, amylaceous diet produces a constipated state of the bowels. The retention of these starchy matters for an undue time in the alimentary canal, soon excites fermentative changes, during which large quantities of gaseous products are generated. This fermentative condition goes on increasing from day to day till the contents of the alimentary canal become one fermentative mass of yeast, when the constipated condition gives way to the irritant cathartic influence of the developing yeast plants and constantly increasing gaseous products: profuse discharges of fecal matters and wind result. Previous to this, however, the fermentation during the constipated stage has — by its irritative influence — produced a peculiar abnormal condition in the follicles of the large intestines and stomach.

Simultaneous with this follicular enlargement is the development of quantities of colloid matter. The intestinal canal and stomach become coated with a pultaceous, yeasty, adherent, offensive matter which excites fermentation in amylaceous food soon after it is eaten. Food taken during the day begins to ferment actively by evening, and the bowels and stomach become distended with gases, continuing so until the food of the day has all been evacuated, when the flatulence gradually disappears. This daily increasing fermentation produces daily increasing irritation, resulting in a constant accession of diarrhœa, which soon assumes a chronic form.

XIX.

THE STOMACH AND BOWELS, AS WE FIND THEM IN CON-
SUMPTION.

THE stomach and bowels, in consumption, are filled with alcoholic and vinegar yeast, and often, in addition, contain butyric acid ferment and the vegetations which excite putrefactive
decomposition in animal matters.

These organs are constantly filled with these yeast plants and
the various products which are formed by the development of
these vegetations, to wit : alcohol, vinegar, carbonic acid, butyric acid, sulphide of ammonium, sulphide of hydrogen and many
other poisonous and deleterious products.

These being continually present, the epithelial surfaces gradually become enervated and so paralyzed by them, that they lose,
little by little, those beautiful and wisely bestowed selective
powers found in healthy states, (by virtue of which only such
products as are required to nourish and maintain the tissues
are taken up,) and begin to "gobble" up the good and the
bad together, — that is, the nutrient matters mixed with these
deleterious yeast vegetations and the products made by their
development.

These vegetations and their situation, together with the deleterious products formed by their multiplication and development, cause all forms of consumptive troubles, whether they
occur in the bowels as chronic diarrhœa; in the lungs either as
tubercular deposits or connective tissue ; increase and shrinkage
of the tubes and alveolar structure from partial paralysis of the
parts, or in any other tissue or organ.

In consumption, the stomach and bowels are "yeast pots."

This is eminently true in all cases, except in instances where the strong accessory causes (either of constitutional syphilis or gravel) invade the lung tissue : the former attacks the mucous membranes and fibrous tissues, while the latter calcifies the trachea and bronchial tubes to a greater or lesser extent. Even in these cases yeast plays a more or less important part in advancing and hastening the final issue. These are the most obstinate cases of consumption to handle that we ever meet with, requiring patient and long-continued medication and diet.

XX.

CONDITION OF THE DIAPHRAGM IN CONSUMPTION.

EARLY in the disease, the diaphragm becomes more or less paralyzed from the gradual absorption of carbonic acid gas from the stomach, which is constantly filled with this gas to a greater or lesser extent.

This partial paralysis of the diaphragm begins in the first part, or incubative stage of the disease, and gradually increases as the disease progresses.

As soon as this organ loses its normal vigor, the abnormal breathing begins and the patient complains of not being fully satisfied with the amount of air entering the lungs; in consequence he every little while draws a long but involuntary breath, elevating the shoulders in so doing. This frequent and deep breathing is called "sighing," and always indicates a partial paralysis of the diaphragm. This paralysis is often excessive, coming on suddenly towards evening or during the night, or sometimes after a full meal of fermenting foods, and produces a feeling of suffocation, constant gasping and a fear of dying.

These spells alarm the patient and friends. They are not as dangerous as they appear. The sufferer, while insisting that he or she cannot breathe, will talk or scream quite as loudly as when well.

If, however, this partial paralysis extends to the heart, the limbs become cold and clammy, the nails and lips blue, and there is now more than seeming danger. The remedy is to stimulate and get the wind out of the stomach as quickly as possible. Hot drinks, stimulants and carminatives are always useful. In extreme cases, ether should be freely used in connection with the hot drinks. Relief comes as soon as the carbonic acid gas is eructated or passed.

XXI.

CONDITION OF THE HEART IN CONSUMPTION.

THE heart is one of the first organs to feel the inroads of consumption. The cardiac end of the stomach rises in its upper wall, above the plane where the œsophagus enters. In this elevated position — which becomes more elevated and distended in a partially paralyzed stomach — the carbonic acid gas gathers above the liquid and solid contents of the organ, and is gradually absorbed. This gas being directly under the heart, that organ soon begins to feel its paralyzing influence. When the cardiac end of the stomach is filled with gas which the patient cannot eructate, (even after taking stimulants, hot drinks and carminatives,) if he will lie down upon the left side, the liquid contents of the stomach will fill the cardiac end and the wind will rise towards the pyloric extremity. This simple device will frequently enable the patient to eructate and pass the gas.

Frequently, in this disease, the patient dies suddenly and long before the lung trouble has rendered death necessary, simply from carbonic acid paralysis of the heart. This usually occurs after a large meal of fermentable and indigestible food. The patient is seized with a sudden coldness; the fingers and lips become blue; the respiration short or oppressed, the lungs often filling up (when the paralysis extends to the lungs) with a tough, tenacious mucus which chokes them if he is unable to expectorate it, and he expires from suffocation.

The inhalation of ether, or of nitrite of amyl, and internal doses of ether at such times will often aid in carrying the patient over the dangerous moment and save life.

XXII.

CONDITION OF THE AIR-PASSAGES IN CONSUMPTION.

THE partial paralysis of the nerves of the throat, trachea and bronchiæ, together with that of the muscles of respiration, is a frequent and serious complication in consumption.

This paralysis is often so complete that patients for months, and sometimes years before death, are unable to speak or cough above a whisper. The throat, fauces and larynx have a scalded feeling and frequently swallowing is very painful and difficult.

There is a sensation as of severe inflammation of the throat and fauces, but on examination the surfaces are found to be pale and anemic, and the parts more dead than alive. The parts are, in truth, partially dead; the scalded feeling comes from this semi-death and is neuralgic. Instead of using the remedies for inflammatory states, as the feelings of the patient and the first impressions of the physician might indicate, those for partially dead and dying tissue should be resorted to. Something should be used to restore life, to increase action and invigorate, rather than to deplete and lessen vitality.

This same half dead condition extends to all parts of the respiratory apparatus, rendering expectoration difficult and ineffective. Even where the voice and cough are strong, the organs of the chest are all more or less paralyzed, and remedial efforts should always take the direction of restoring tone to the parts, and of preventing the useless expenditure of what little vital energy remains to these organs.

The patient should rest: much talking and fatiguing exercise should be prohibited. All exercise should be passive, such as rubbing, careful kneading and driving in an easy carriage. All excitements, worries, excessive mental efforts and physical exertions should be avoided. The life should be as calm, passive and happy as possible.

XXIII.

GRAVEL OF THE LUNGS, MELANOTIC MATTER, AND GIANT
CELLS. THE RELATIONS THEY BEAR TO EACH OTHER AND
TO CONSUMPTION AS ACCESSORIES, NOT CAUSES.

MELANOTIC matter never is formed, I believe, in the lungs, except in cases of gravel of these organs. The melanotic matter always accompanies the formation of gravelly matter in the pulmonary tissue, and the gravel never occurs without its melanotic accompaniment.

The so-called " *Giant Cells* " are the necessary consequence of the formation, in the bronchial membranes, of insoluble particles of unorganized and sometimes of organic matter.

These " *Giant Cells* " are a provision of Nature to carry insoluble matters out of the follicles and parent cells.

The giant cell membranes form around the melanotic and gravelly granules, and serve as vehicles for transporting them out of the parent cells and follicles, and finally out of the organism.

Gravel of the lungs is the secondary cause of asthma in all its forms; the preliminary cause being that peculiar diseased or deranged state of digestion and assimilation — the result of unhealthy alimentation — which eventuates in this gravel.

Gravel of the lungs often precedes and accompanies consumption, complicating and aggravating the disease, and rendering it more difficult and tedious to cure.

These complicated cases are known, in common parlance, as slow, or fibrous consumption. A bronchial cough often precedes this form of the disease by many years.

This form is known as fibrous consumption (Pulmonary Fibrosis), because the fibrous structure of the bronchiæ and their lining mucous membranes, are often, and in fact always more or less thickened and are frequently filled with gravelly particles ; sometimes also the larynx and bronchi are so calcified that they have the appearance of long tubes.

In such instances the patients lose their voices many months before death, and frequently die suddenly while yet they have considerable strength — during a paroxysm of strangling cough.

When the gravelly diathesis establishes itself in lungs which are not yet affected by the specific cause of consumption, consumption cannot be produced by it. But when the specific cause is either already in operation, or sets in afterwards, it hastens the progress of the disease and complicates it.

In this way constitutional syphilis, when it attacks the pulmonary mucous membranes in a consumptive patient, accelerates the disease and renders the case much more formidable to handle, and the hope of success more remote, as both causes have to be met and combated.

The same may be said when there is gravel of the lungs, with a tendency to calcification of the bronchial tubes.

The latter cases, although slow in progress, are more difficult to handle than simple cases wherein the specific cause of consumption is alone operative.

XXIV.

PULMONARY FIBROSIS, OR FIBROUS CONSUMPTION.

THIS is a disease arising from the over-development and hardening of the fibrous or connective tissue of the lungs, which pathological condition and state is here indicated as pulmonary fibrosis, — fibrous consumption or slow consumption. It is usually accompanied by gravel of the lungs, is of long continuance and slow progress.

To the ordinary observer it begins and continues for a long time as what appears to be simply a bronchial catarrh.

It may or may not be attended with asthmatic symptoms. It may later on be hastened in its progress by the formation of tubercular deposits, though often it is quite free from this complication. The lungs shrink and harden, and the power of dilating and contracting them becomes less and less under the control of the patient, the lung tissues and all the muscles of respiration continually and gradually becoming more and more paralyzed.

The secretion from the mucous membrane is more or less tough, ropy, stringy and adhesive. This secretion may be made in greater or lesser quantities, according to the extent of the paralysis of the parts at the time, and the amount of irritation arising from colds, gravel and other causes of bronchial irritation.

In the earlier stages the voice is more or less husky and hoarse. As the disease advances the hoarseness and huskiness increase, till in many instances the voice is lost, — talking and coughing being mostly a whisper and breath cough.

This form of the disease occurs where the patient lives almost entirely upon fermentable food, and the fermentative processes have for a long time remained chiefly confined to the stomach and have not passed downward into the small and large intestines to any great extent. The products of fermentation, and especially the carbonic acid gas, are gradually absorbed in daily increasing quantity, till the diaphragm and intercostal muscles, and the heart and the connective and mucous tissues of the lungs become so paralyzed that the lungs are but partially dilated during inspiration, and the circulation is in consequence imperfect, there being a stasis or stagnant state in the blood apparatus of the parts.

In this state of low vitalization, the glue and mucous tissues at first thicken and are over-fed, by virtue of which the same kind of growth, development and thickening, and the same viscid secretion of mucus occurs as takes place in the large intestines in consumption of the bowels. Later on in the disease, the blood becomes so poor that even this stasis in the circulation of the parts is unable to supply them with sufficient nourishment to keep pace with the waste, and the hardened and thickened parts now shrink and become more and more useless, occupying less and less space.

The whole body becomes extremely emaciated; the patient becomes often voiceless and coughs and speaks in a faint breath, and finally expires from tissue exhaustion and starvation.

In pulmonary fibrosis we have an increase and consolidation of the interlobular connective tissue, with a cellular infiltration and thickening of the alveolar walls. These two histological changes are characteristic of this form of disease. In connection with these changes we have an accumulation of yeasty and epithelial products within the pulmonary alveoli, which is common to the tubercular form of the disease. The paralysis of the pulmonary tissues, larynx, fauces and muscles of respiration is much more pronounced in pulmonary fibrosis than it is in tubercular consumption. Whenever tubercular deposits occur in this form of consumption, they are found in the alveoli and alveolar walls, and rarely in the connective tissues and capillaries.

Gravelly or calcified deposits are often formed in the pulmonary membranes and bronchial connective tissue: in fact, the tracheal and bronchial tubes become sometimes completely calcified.

The same primary cause is the basis of both these forms of disease.

The differences between pulmonary fibrosis and tubercular consumption, so far as the cause is concerned, consist in the location and manner of the attack and the operation of the cause.

In pulmonary fibrosis, acid yeasts for the most part develop in and remain in the stomach, the pyloric valve keeping a close watch to prevent their passage into the small bowels to any great extent. In consequence of this, the acid yeasts have not the opportunity of gaining access to the blood stream in a quantity sufficient to form emboli for blocking up the pulmonary capillaries. In tubercular consumption, on the contrary, the acid yeasts are constantly passing through the stomach into the small bowels, where they are swiftly taken up with the food and pass into the blood stream, there accumulating as emboli.

As soon as these emboli become too large to pass freely through the constantly expanding and contracting lung capillaries, these vessels act as a filter to the blood, gathering up the largest plugs, which now dam up the vessels and form nuclei for tubercles.

The reason why these emboli are usually caught first in the upper lobes of the lungs, is that the cold air first enters these parts, and becomes gradually warmed before reaching the lower lobes.

The colder the air, the more it contracts the connective tissue, and this contraction lessens the size of the capillary vessels just enough to make of the upper lobes a little finer sieve than the lower.

The thickening in the alveolar walls and the increase in the interlobular connective tissue in pulmonary fibrosis is not, strictly speaking, owing to an inflammatory process. It is a condition and result of partial paralysis, or partial death, or a lowering of the vital energy of the parts from causes that paralyze partially, and would paralyze to the extent of producing entire death of the parts, if the degree of exposure were sufficiently increased.

It is a painless process, a partial death resulting in a stasis of the blood vessels and stream, which causes a damming up of the blood, or an accumulated lingering in the stream, resulting in hypernutrition and a thickened, gluey and more or less abundant secretion of mucus [1] from the alveolar walls, which blocks up and congests the cells and follicles. By virtue of this process, nutrition and organization of a low type ensue, and imperfectly organized tissue is formed. This is simply hypertrophy of tissue without extravasation, a condition similar to that which occurs in thickening of the colon in chronic diarrhœa (or consumption of the bowels), or that which exists in ovarian or goitrous developments, and in the formation of uterine fibroids and other fibrous growths and thickenings. It is hypernutrition from partial paralysis of the parts, resulting in a stasis of the blood flow — or a lingering in the nutrient blood stream — from which arises an excessive and imperfect formation of a tissue too poorly and incompletely organized to possess much vitality and endurance: in consequence this tissue is destined to have but a brief existence before it begins to break down or to disintegrate in some way.

Figs. 1, 2, 3 and 4, Plate XVI, represent the ciliated cells shed from the bronchial membranes.

Fig. 3, same plate, represents a large mucous cell just escaping from a ciliated cell.

---

[1] When the nerves of a mucous membrane become partially paralyzed through an injury, or from the absorption of carbonic acid gas, or from any other cause, immediately a secretion of thick, ropy, gluey mucus is poured out. This mucus is often so sticky and thick that it blocks up the follicles of the parts and produces a congestion proportional to the degree of paralysis.

Fig. 4, Plate XVI, represents a ciliated cell filled and much distended with mucous cells.

Figs. 5, 6, 7, 10, 13, 17, 18, 25, 26, 31, 32 and 54, Plate XVI, represent giant cells of the various types, some filled with albuminoid granules, and others containing, in addition to these, granules of gravel and melanotic matter.

Figs. 14, 23, 24, 27, 28, 29, 34, 35, 36, 37, 38, Plate XVI, represent crystals, calculi and granules of oxalate of lime and cystine in the sputa, where the fibrous consumption is complicated with asthma.

Figs. 39, 40, 41, 42, 44, 45, 46, 47, Plate XVII, represent calculi, crystals and granules of gravel in the sputa of fibrous consumption, with asthmatic complications.

Fig. 1, Plate XIII, represents the appearance of the blood in fibrous consumption, in an advanced stage of the disease. The blood is ropy and thin, and the fibrin filaments strongly marked, from the fact that the filaments are short and thickened, — which increases the size of the meshes formed by the filaments. This fine meshwork obstructs the free flow of the globules, hence the ropiness. This is caused by the long-continued souring of foods in the stomach and in the absorption of the acid formed.

XXV.

YEAST VEGETATIONS OFTEN DEVELOPING DURING CONSUMP-
TION, IN THE SKIN — EITHER OVER PORTIONS OR OVER
THE ENTIRE SURFACE OF THE BODY — AND IN THE MUCOUS
MEMBRANES OF THE DIGESTIVE ORGANS AND AIR PASSAGES.

OFTEN in the later stages of consumption, especially after
the night sweats begin, alcoholic and acid yeasts are found
developing in vast quantities in the outer layer of the skin,
over the entire surface of the body and in the mucous membranes generally.

These vegetations are represented at Figs. 1, 2, 3, 4, 5, 6, 7,
8, 9, 10, 11, 12, 13, 14, 15, 16, 17, 18, 19, 20, 21, 22, 23,
Plate XIV ; 24, 25, 26, 27, 28, 29, 30, 31, 32, 33, 34, 35, 36,
37, 38, 39 and 40, Plate XV ; 55, Plate XIV ; 61, 62, 63, 64,
66, 67, 68, 69, 70, 71, 72, 73, 74, 75, 76 and 77, Plate XV.
Figs. 17, 19, 20, 21, 22, 24, Plate XIV, and 66 Plate XV, represent the same vegetation separated from the epidermic cells.

The other vegetations occur in the mucous membranes and
secretions of the lungs and digestive organs.

When these vegetations are rapidly developing upon these
surfaces, the tendency to chills, fevers and sweats is marked,
the perspiration is more or less profuse, sour and often very
exhausting. The cold stage usually comes on at or before noon
and lasts from half an hour to two hours. This is followed by
the hot febrile stage, which usually continues to a greater or
lesser degree until after bedtime.

The hot stage is terminated by a profuse, cold perspiration,
which may last most of the night and is often very debilitating.

Occasionally in excessive vegetable and cereal feeders, this
yeast vegetation develops in patches on the chest, neck and

arms, producing brown, slightly raised spots from one-fourth to several inches in diameter. The epidermis becomes thickened, soft, spongy and raised, and is easily scraped off. The vegetation has received the names Trichophyton Furfur and Microsporon Furfur.

XXVI.

TUBERCLE.

The consumptive deposits which have received the name of tubercle have nothing to do as a cause of the disease, but are simply deposits formed by the specific cause, which may take place under the proper conditions.

They are caused by little emboli of either Mycoderma spores, alone or coupled with adhesive, colorless corpuscles, and sticky fibrin. The Mycoderma spores may accumulate either in the follicles and epithelial surfaces of the minute bronchi and air cells; outside of the air cells, in the connective tissue; or in and blocking up the capillary vessels that envelop and surround the air cells. The more acute and rapid the disease, the more the deposits are found in the mucous surfaces and follicles, and in the capillaries. The slower it progresses, the more the deposits involve the fibrous tissues, producing what is known in common parlance as " slow consumption."

This slow form of the disease is determined by the presence of an anterior disease — gravel of the lungs — which has produced in the patient for months, and often for years previous to the advent of the consumptive phase, a bronchial cough and catarrh.

This gravelly disease retards the progress of the consumptive cause.

Whether the deposits take place in the air cells, alveolar walls, interlobular tissue or pulmonary capillaries, they are all produced by the same general cause, and tend to the same general result. All animals and men in the state of nature — or when they are provided with the food that they were constructed and constituted to digest well — are free from consumptive diseases. These only occur in domesticated and partially domesticated animals, and among the so-called civilized and partially civilized human beings, when they are deprived of their natural food, or when they become victims of unhealthy alimentation.

There appears to be in civilization a tendency to constantly court the cravings of diseased and unnaturally cultivated tastes, appetites and desires, taking small heed of the ability of the organism to digest and assimilate. The result is all that such unnatural doings could lead us to expect, and we have from unhealthy feeding a death rate which is truly appalling. In this country alone, aside from the multitudes dying of paralysis, softening of the brain, insanity, heart disease, rheumatism, ovarian disease, cancers, Bright's disease, diabetes, etc., we have over twenty-five thousand deaths from consumption annually.

All of this is but a just retribution for physical sins, or yielding to the cravings and longings of cultivated and diseased appetites and desires.

That deposit which in consumption is called tubercle, is simply a local and later manifestation of a general systemic cause, which has been in operation for some time before the physical signs of this condition of the disease have shown themselves. The stage precedent to the deposit of tubercles is of greater or lesser duration, and varies with the diet, exercise, constitution and the natural strength or weakness of certain bodily organs. It is characterized by specific conditions and symptoms which gradually increase in intensity as the disease progresses. There are four stages in the life history of consumption.

First or Incubative Stage.

In the first stage the specific cause is entirely confined to and in the digestive apparatus.

Second or Stage of Transmission.

In the second stage the specific cause is being transmitted from the digestive organs to the blood glands and stream.

Third or Formative Stage.

In the third stage the specific cause has so accumulated in masses or emboli in the blood stream, that these emboli of yeast spores begin to get too large to float freely through the pulmonary capillary vessels, in consequence of which they are caught and held, forming nuclei for tubercles.

Fourth or Stage of Interstitial Death, Softening and Disintegration.

In the fourth stage the tubercular deposits begin to break down, and interstitial death and disintegration begin to go on. This state of things ushers in chills, fevers and sweats.

XXVII.

WHY TUBERCULAR DEPOSITS ARE MORE APT TO OCCUR IN LUNG TISSUE THAN ELSEWHERE.

IT is under a most wise provision that we are fitted with elastic organs like the lungs, the tissues and capillaries of which are subject to expansion and contraction from the hot and cold air we breathe.

This makes the lung capillaries smaller, as a rule, than those of any other part of the body. They are thus enabled to act as filters to the blood, gathering up all the particles, masses and emboli that are too large to float safely through the brain and other highly vitalized but less elastic parts.

This is the reason why the small masses of mycoderma spores are caught and held in the lungs, forming there nuclei for tubercles, and also why the lungs are more liable to become involved in tubercular consumption than are our other organs. Some animals — the rabbit and guinea pig, for example — are so sensitive in these parts that no matter what is thrown into the blood stream, if it should happen to form a blood clot there, tubercular disease of the lungs is sure to follow.

For this reason these animals are not suitable ones with which to experiment in this disease.

XXVIII.

WHY TUBERCULAR DEPOSITS ARE MORE LIABLE TO TAKE
PLACE IN THE UPPER, THAN IN THE LOWER LOBES OF THE
LUNGS.

IT is well known that tubercular deposits are much more
liable to occur in the upper lobes of the lungs than in the
lower.

The reason of this is that the upper lobes are first exposed to
the cold air on inhaling, and become more contracted in consequence than are the lower portions which receive the air later
on and after it has become somewhat warmer.

The lungs are elastic organs composed largely of elastic and
non-elastic connective tissue, which tissue is very sensitive to
changes in temperature, and contracts and expands with heat
and cold. The contraction narrows the capillary vessels; on
this account the parts first receiving the air are more contracted
than are the parts lower down, and the capillaries in consequence become a finer sieve just there and hence catch such
emboli as can easily pass through those of other parts of the
body.

In infancy, before we are exposed to outside cold air, the
tendency for tubercular deposits to localize in the upper part of
the lungs, is not so great. At this early period the meningeal
membranes are more in danger than the lung tissue.

XXIX.

COUGH AND SPUTUM IN CONSUMPTION.

DURING the first and second stages of consumption there is not necessarily any cough or expectoration, yet both of these are present in many cases, from catarrhs and bronchial irritations.

The catarrhs may have become established from continually taking cold, as persons living almost exclusively upon fermenting food are liable to do, on account of the alcoholic, vinegar and carbonic acid products constantly passing off through the air passages, which keeps the pores partially paralyzed, open and enervated.

Deranged digestion and assimilation also frequently result in a gravelly diathesis, which manifests itself by the formation of granular and crystalline particles, and small calculi in the mucous follicles of the air passages, and later on in the connective tissue of the bronchial tubes and trachea and larynx, wherever there is any irritation of an enervated, paralytic type.

Whenever there is expectoration in the first two stages (the pretubercular stage), the sputum is usually clear, viscid and jelly-like: when gravel is present it takes on a grayish and bluish cast, being very tough, ropy and full of giant cells, many of which are filled with granular gravel covered with melanotic matter. This sputum also contains many granules, crystals and often small calculi, outside of giant cells.

With the advent of the third stage, cough and expectoration of the real consumptive type begin.

The sputum is at first quite clear and viscid, but soon becomes more opaque and filled with the spores of the mycoderms. The vegetation is most abundant in cases that are progressing most rapidly. In pure consumption there are no giant cells and gravel in the sputa. These only occur when the disease is complicated with bronchial catarrhs and gravel of the lungs. Throughout this stage the sputum is ropy and viscid, and free from connective tissue shreds. There is no interstitial death and disintegration of lung tissue.

The fourth stage is ushered in by chills, fevers and sweats, and with sputum containing a greater or lesser quantity of shreds of disintegrating connective tissue, caused by interstitial death and decay and by the softening and breaking down of tubercular deposits.

The shreds are of both elastic and non-elastic connective tissue fibre.

The presence of these shreds in the sputa always marks the presence of the fourth or breaking-down stage, and as long as the dying and disintegration continue, the chills, fevers and sweats continue also, and the disease progresses.

The condition in this stage is that the death and decay of tissue is more rapid than the repair : in other words, the system is not sufficiently nourished. Food is not digested and assimilated so as to make blood fast enough to repair the waste which is going on.

What is wanted now is more blood to make more tissue, that the repair may be greater than the waste.

As soon as this is accomplished, the chills, fevers and sweats cease ; the cough and expectoration begin to subside, and the patient is on the road to health. This road is necessarily a long and tedious one, but the route is safe and sure.

XXX.

PRECAUTIONARY MEASURES FOR PREVENTING AND CHECKING HEMORRHAGE.

In consumption there always exists — in variable extent — a softened condition of the glue or connective tissue.

It is this tissue which makes up the ropes, cords, strings, threads and bands, sheaths and membranes which tie, support, hold together and maintain in place all the tissues and organs of the body, and the tubes of the blood-vessels, of the respiratory apparatus and digestive organs, etc., etc. This tissue holds every part of us together and in place, and conveys all materials into and out of the body. Although not a highly vitalized tissue, it makes up a large percentage of our framework, and is of the greatest consequence in giving support and strength, and for supplying the avenues to, into and out of all parts of the organism. This is the tissue in which nearly all pathological growths occur.

When this tissue becomes softened by unhealthy feeding, as it does in this disease, the whole machine begins to weaken and lose its power of endurance.

The fibrous sheaths of the blood-vessels are liable to become ruptured during excitements and over-exertions. The mental excitement of troubled dreams often ruptures them. Hence the importance of using all the means in our power to provide against this danger, and, when the danger has come, to prevent serious and fatal results. The first and most important consideration is to stop all excitements, over-exertions and all unhealthy feeding; stop the use of all foods that are fermenting in the stomach and bowels, and employ only those aliments that can be well digested. In connection with this the stomach should be washed out from one to two hours before meals and half an hour before retiring, with warm water or clear, weak tea. This course will improve digestion and assimilation; reparative blood will be made, and all the tissues will begin the process of reconstruction. The repair of worn-out, partially dead and softened tissues takes time.

Accidents may occur during this period, so that it is necessary to be on our guard, and to use the best means at hand for preventing the rupture of blood-vessels.

As a precautionary measure, if the bowels are not too loose, administer a small dose — from an eighth (⅛) to a teaspoonful of Epsom salts in the hot water one hour before breakfast, and take from half to a teaspoonful of either the Fluid Extract of Witch Hazel, or the bark of the Apple Tree Root in a little water two hours after each meal. The bowels should be moved once daily and the whole system kept in the most perfect order.

If at any time bleeding should occur, inhale with the atomizer a solution of one dram of Liquor Ferri Persulphatis in eight ounces of water. This should be deeply and freely inhaled whenever there are any signs of bleeding. Inhale as often as is necessary to keep the broken vessels plugged up, and continue the inhalation each time from three to four minutes, or until the bleeding is thoroughly checked.

Keep perfectly passive and quiet, avoiding all excitement, conversation and company. Keep a recumbent posture, with the head and body raised at an angle of about 45°, till the vessels are thoroughly healed. During the hemorrhages keep up the Epsom salts and take one of the Fluid Extracts before named. The atomizer, already filled and prepared, should stand always at hand to use at a moment's notice.

By employing these precautions, bleeding at the lungs will be a rare occurrence, and when it does happen it will do but little harm.

XXXI.

OBJECT OF DRINKING HOT WATER ONE OR MORE HOURS BEFORE MEALS, AND HALF AN HOUR BEFORE RETIRING.

THE digestive organs in consumption may be aptly compared to an old vinegar barrel, and like it, they require frequent and thorough washing out before any fermentable food can be taken in without fermenting.   This washing should be done by drinking hot water at about 110° Fahr. and should take place long enough before each meal to allow the water and washings to get out of the stomach before the food is eaten, and to keep ahead of the food as it passes down the stomach and bowels. From experience I find that this hot-water washing should not be nearer the meal than one hour, and it is often better to set back the time to two hours.   From fifteen to thirty minutes should be taken for drinking the water, so that the stomach may not be uncomfortably distended.

The object of the hot water is to wash out a dirty, yeasty, slimy, sour stomach before eating and sleeping.   It should be taken on retiring, in order that the stomach may be as clean as possible to sleep upon and may not excite troubled sleep, dreams or wakefulness: also to prevent fermenting products from lying over night next the diaphragm, heart and lungs, partially paralyzing them and exciting cough, or disturbing the breathing and circulation.

It is necessary to continue this washing regularly and to keep it up with persistence for months and even for years, before the digestive apparatus becomes so thoroughly cleansed of yeast plants and the products developed by their growth, as to allow normal digestion without the aid of hot water.   The water should be taken as above prescribed in every case of any disease, and forms an inseparable and invaluable adjunct to this radical method of cure. It is in fact seldom that a person is found possessed of sufficiently good digestion as to render this washing useless. It quenches thirst more effectually than any other drink and acts as a gentle stimulant to all the organs in their performance of their normal functions.

It is better to take the hot water in the morning while in bed, or if up, to lie down on the left side after taking it. This position allows a freer passage to the wind and gases which the hot water helps to eructate. The best times for taking it are at about six a. m., eleven a. m., four p. m. and nine p. m. It is not alone in consumption that this practice of drinking hot water is of use, but in all diseases arising from defective digestive processes and from the fermentation of foods. Even comparatively healthy persons find it of much benefit. It excites downward peristalsis, dilutes the ropy secretions of the body, dissolves all abnormal crystalline substances that may be present in the blood and urine, and everywhere promotes elimination. It supplies a foundation for the thorough treatment of all chronic diseases by an inside bath which cleanses and refreshes the entire system. Cold water cannot take its place. It was at first tried in connection with food experiments and found to cause pain and colic : it does not assist in the eructation of gas produced by fermentation, because it does not excite downward peristalsis of the alimentary canal, as does water at a temperature of 110° to 150° Fahr., such as is liked in drinking tea or coffee. The common and excessive use of cold water, both in drinking and bathing, is a very great mistake. It depresses the system and wastes the animal heat in the effort to restore the temperature of the economy which is sensibly lowered by it, and the nerve force needed by the various organs, of which we have none too much at any time, is draughted off to repair our mistake. When we ice our water, we intensify this error an hundred-fold, and sacrifice the well-being of all internal organs, for the temporary cooling of mouth and throat. If those surfaces were in perfectly normal condition, we should not crave this cooling; this taste, like the appetite for liquors, wines and drinks of all description, is a cultivated and abnormal one. Such have no place in the healthy system; they are symptoms of disease and warn us of a subbasic cause which must be removed. I have known confirmed drunkards, after they have been kept from all spirituous liquors and cured of diseased appetites by the restoration of tone to the digestive apparatus, to admit that they preferred hot water to liquor in any form, and to keep it up throughout life as a stimulant to digestion.

Lukewarm water has also been tried, but was found to excite upward peristalsis and to make the men sick at the stomach. It was only after repeated experiments that the most favorable temperature, amount and hours for taking the hot water were determined accurately as above given.

XXXII.

DRINKS, FOOD, BATHS, EXERCISE AND CLOTHING ADVISABLE IN CONSUMPTION.

Drinks. — Drink from half a pint to a pint of hot water, from one to two hours before each meal and on retiring, for the purpose of washing out the slimy, yeasty and bilious stomach before eating and sleeping.

Drink a cup of clear tea, coffee or beef tea (the latter free from fat), towards the close of each meal, sipping slowly. During the interval, between two hours after, and one hour before each meal, drink hot water or beef tea if thirsty.

Food Meats. — Eat the muscle pulp of lean beef made into cakes and broiled. This pulp should be as free as possible from connective or glue tissue, fat and cartilage. The " American Chopper " answers very well for separating the connective tissue, this being driven down in front of the knife to the bottom of the board. In chopping, the beef should not be stirred up in the chopper, but the muscle pulp should be scraped off with a spoon at intervals during the chopping. At the end of the chopping, the fibrous tissue of the meat (the portion which makes up fibrous growths) all lies on the bottom board of the chopper. This may be utilized as soup meat for well people.

Previous to chopping, the fat, bones, tendons and fasciæ should all be cut away, and the lean muscle cut up in pieces an inch or two square. Steaks cut through the centre of the round are the richest and best for this purpose. Beef should be procured from well fatted animals that are from four to six years old.

The pulp should not be pressed too firmly together before

broiling, or it will taste livery. Simply press it sufficiently to hold it together. Make the cakes from half an inch to an inch thick. Broil slowly and moderately well over a fire free from blaze and smoke. When cooked, put it on a hot plate and season to taste with butter, pepper and salt; also use either Worcestershire or Halford sauce, mustard, horseradish or lemon juice on the meat if desired. Celery may be moderately used as a relish. No other meats should be allowed till the stomach becomes clean, the urine uniformly clear and free, standing at a density of from 1.015–1.020, and the cough and expectoration so improved that they cease to be troublesome. When this time arrives, bring in for variety as side dishes, broiled lamb, broiled mutton, broiled game, broiled chicken, oysters broiled or roasted in the shell, boiled codfish (fresh or salt), broiled and baked fish free from fat, and broiled dried beef, chipped thin and sprinkled over broiled beefsteak to give it a relish. A soft boiled egg may be taken at breakfast occasionally with the meat if it does not heighten the color of the urine.

Bread. — Bread, toast, boiled rice or cracked wheat may be eaten in the proportion of one part (by bulk) to from four to six parts of the meat. The bread should be free from sugar and raised with yeast. It may be made from gluten flour, white flour or Graham flour; corn meal preparations should be avoided.

All things not previously enumerated and the following articles of food in especial should not be eaten, viz.: beans, soups, sweets, pies, cakes, pickles, sauce, preserves, fruits, vegetables, greens, pancakes, fritters, crullers, griddle-cakes and mush. Vinegar should be carefully avoided.

Baths. — Take a soap and hot-water bath twice a week for cleanliness, after which oil the entire body with glycerine and water, rubbing in well. Every night sponge body and limbs with one quart of hot water, in which put from one to four teaspoonfuls of aqua ammonia, after which rub well and wipe dry. Every morning sponge off with a little hot water, wiping dry and rubbing thoroughly. Avoid washing in cold water, that there may be no unnecessary expenditure of nervous force in the restoration of vital warmth to chilled surfaces. Our constant endeavor must be to preserve and increase the store of vital energy, and no steps in this direction, however small apparently, are unimportant ones.

Clothing. — Wear flannel next the skin and dress with comfortable warmth. Change all clothing worn during the day on retiring, so that it may be thoroughly aired for the following morning. Keep the clothing sweet and clean by changing every other day.

Exercise. — Drive daily in the open air as much as possible without fatigue. If not able to drive, the body and limbs should be rubbed, kneaded and pounded all over for ten minutes, morning, noon and night, by some one who has sufficient strength to do it thoroughly.

Meals. — Meals should be taken at regular intervals, and it is better not to sit down at a table where others are indulging in all kinds of food. Eat alone, or with others who are on the same diet. After the system gets in good running order, which is indicated by the urine flowing at the rate of from three pints to two quarts in twenty-four hours, and standing constantly at 1.020 density, the appetite becomes good, and usually more than three meals a day are desired. This desire for food should be gratified by allowing the patient a nice piece of broiled steak, with a cup of clear tea, coffee, hot water or beef tea, midway between the breakfast and dinner, and dinner and supper.

If the directions here given are faithfully followed out and persisted in, consumption *in all its stages* becomes a curable disease.

All anodynes that disorder the stomach are to be rigidly avoided. No medicines of any kind should be taken, except such as are prescribed by a physician. The cure is accomplished by getting the system in splendid basic condition, when the urine becomes clear and flows at the rate of three pints or more

per diem, standing at 1.020 density, the appetite becomes enormous, and from two to four pounds of lean beef are eaten daily.
The chills, fevers and sweats, growing lighter, soon cease entirely. Blood-making processes go on rapidly; the blood-vessels
fill out; repair of tissues begins and steadily continues; the eyes
brighten; the cough lessens by degrees; interstitial death, decay
and disintegration of lung tissue cease; the entire organism is
pervaded by the glow of health, and step by step the patient (if
he perseveres) advances safely and surely towards the goal of
cure, to reach which, only patience and the strict observance
of the rules here laid down are required. To accomplish this
end, both diet and treatment are to be minutely and conscien-
tiously carried out in all their details, with the soul and body of
the patient firmly enlisted in the good cause. All this of course
takes time, for it is Nature, after all, that does the work. Consequently all the changes must be physiological, and as such
can only ensue as rapidly as the human machine — when well
run — can organize and repair.

The physician must know precisely what to do, and do it. He
must watch his patient daily, scrutinize excretions, secretions
and blood alike carefully, and see that every part of the pro-
gramme is faithfully and honestly carried out. Any deviation
from the right course can be at once detected by increased fermentation ; the consequent biliousness ; heightened color of
urine ; aggravation of cough, and all the other pathological
symptoms. Patients cannot deceive the physician skilled in
this field of positive work. If the directions are all rigidly followed, the machine will soon get to running nicely and continue
to do so unless thrown off the track by deviations. Such departures should be at once detected and corrected, or the patient
begins to lose ground.

No one need hope to handle consumption successfully by
change of climate or by medicinal remedies. It is a disease arising from long-continued, unhealthy alimentation, and can only
be cured by the removal of its cause. This cause is fermenting

food, and the products of this fermentation (carbonic acid gas, alcoholic and vinegar yeast and vinegar) are the more important factors in developing the peculiar pathological symptoms, conditions and states in this complaint, which is generally and erroneously believed to be incurable.

Consumption of the bowels can be produced at any time in the human subject, in from fifteen to thirty days, and consumption of the lungs within three months, by special, exclusive and continued feeding upon the diet that produces them.

XXXIII.

INFLUENCE OF CLIMATE AND EXERCISE IN CONSUMPTION OF THE BOWELS.

It has been noticed that there is a greater liability to consumption of the bowels (chronic diarrhœa), in warm malarious regions than in the non-malarious: from this fact has arisen a prevalent belief that the malady is a miasmatic one. In all malarious regions there is a much greater tendency to the development of low cryptogamic forms, while fermentation is sooner excited and progresses more energetically than in non-malarious localities. This increased tendency in malarious districts to the development of yeast and other cryptogamic plants, and consequently to the development of fermentative changes, will undoubtedly explain the reason why, in such places, there is an increased liability to consumption of the bowels. In such localities the gelatinous (colloid) products of the feces are peculiarly marked, and seem to aggravate the diarrhœa. The intestines appear to be in a condition to afford a proper nidus for the development of this peculiar matter. It does not, however, appear to have anything to do as an exciting cause of the disease, it being merely a consequence of especial saccharine and fermentative conditions of the system. As soon as these are corrected, colloid matter ceases to develop. In the army, for example, it will always be noticed that the men are much more liable to attacks of diarrhœa during and immediately subsequent to long marches, and after having lived for some time on a dry amylaceous diet which has produced more or less constipation, than they are when situated so that they may cook, and feed plenteously upon good meat and vegetables.

This form of diarrhœa is always preceded and accompanied by active fermentative changes in the alimentary canal, developing large quantities of gaseous products attended with eructations which are generally more or less sour. The disease is very apt to run into a chronic form if not taken early in hand.

In the early stages of the complaint, a simple change of diet from the farinaceous to the albuminous, frequently suffices to cure the disease in a few days. If this cannot be done, a simple cathartic dose of Rochelle salts to clean out the alimentary ferment, followed by small, highly diluted doses of the vegetable acid salts of potassa and iron, will check the disease in the majority of cases. That amylaceous food is the principal cause of chronic diarrhœa is further evidenced by the fact that the officers, who live on more of an albuminous and vegetable diet than the men, and have facilities for carrying and cooking a variety of food, are exempt from the disease, except when they subject themselves to the amylaceous diet of the men. The active fermentation and development of yeast plants, and the resultant gaseous products in the alimentary canal, act as an irritant poison and cathartic of a peculiar character. This is evidenced by the colloid condition which they produce in the stomach and large intestines. They also produce paralytic symptoms in the bowels, extremities, head, and in fact over the whole body. These symptoms are manifested in the involuntary discharges, in numb and pricking sensations in the limbs, the confused, deadened feeling in the head, ringing in the ears, etc.

Carbonic acid, when introduced into the system gradually (in abnormal quantities) by inhalation, has a tendency to produce ringing in the ears; confused, numb sensations in the head, and more or less paralysis of the nerves of sensation and motion.

The gaseous and yeast products also produce bronchial and pulmonary irritation, with a remarkable tendency to tuberculosis, thrombosis and embolism.

XXXIV.

THROMBOSIS AND EMBOLISM FROM THE TOO EXCLUSIVE AND
CONTINUOUS USE OF FOODS AND DRINKS UNDERGOING ACID
FERMENTATION.

THE diseases of which I shall briefly treat in the remaining
chapters of this work, have all of them their primary cause
in unhealthy alimentation, as it is heretofore defined. I shall
in each case indicate the modus operandi of the products of
fermentation, as they vary their point of attack, leaving it to
the intelligent student of this work as a whole, to arrange these
various processes in his mind and sum up their entire effect in
the organism.

We have now to consider that special pathological mode
which results in thrombosis and embolism.

If either animals or men feed too freely upon sour foods and
drinks, which are undergoing or have undergone acid fermentation; or upon foods not yet sour, but sure to become so as soon
as they enter a digestive apparatus already charged with acid
yeasts, the sour products pass more or less rapidly into the circulation, making the blood acid, sticky, ropy and adherent, and
the fibrin filaments tough, larger and shorter. These changes
cause a partial clotting of the blood in the blood stream. This
partial clotting makes the blood mucilaginous, adhesive and
stringy. It also renders the sticky, colorless corpuscles and fibrin
filaments liable to fasten themselves to the walls of the vessels.
The most favorable place for these attachments to take place, is
in or near the heart. They are at first small, consisting of a
few sticky cells and filaments : these minute beginnings grow
by constant additions from the sticky materials of the blood

stream; they become long and flagellate and their growing masses are constantly whipped by the flowing blood stream. The place of attachment is usually small, the mass becoming bellied or fusiform, tapering at both ends and growing more rapidly in the middle. Thrombosis is the name of this condition.

Sooner or later these thrombi are liable to break from their fastenings, when they go floating along in the blood stream as emboli. Now comes in the danger of embolism, or the sudden plugging up of the smaller arterial extremities and capillary vessels.[1] As long as the thrombi remain anchored, or held to their fastenings, there is but little danger of death, although they may produce great discomfort. The more quiet the mental and physical state, the less the danger of tearing them loose. The greater the exertion, the greater the danger.

When they do break loose and block up the capillaries and smaller arterial extremities in any organ, a sudden damming up of the blood in that part takes place, accompanied often by " trip-hammer " pulsations of the heart, effusion of serum, inflammation, and frequently the rupture of blood-vessels in the part or parts, followed by death in from four to forty-eight hours.

This is precisely what occurs in animals and men, when sour foods — too exclusively and continuously eaten — produce too great and rapid acidity of the blood. This often occurs in the disease in swine known as " hog cholera," or consumption of the bowels, and in man sometimes in the so-called chronic diarrhœa, or consumption of the bowels.

Both of these diseases are phases or states which may arise from too rapid infiltration, or saturating the system too quickly and suddenly with acid and acid yeasts. The same foods that produce these states might be taken without serious results, if they could be given in small quantities at first and gradually increased, allowing the various organs to accustom themselves

[1] For examples see chapter on Experiments on Swine.

to caring for and to eliminating the deleterious products, so that they should not accumulate in the system. This mode of taking such foods, combined with proper exercise and surroundings, would maintain a passable condition — though not a healthy one — for a long time.

The foods suited to this condition are those given in the chapter on Uterine Fibroids, together with the general treatment therein indicated.

XXXV.

ASTHMA : ITS CAUSE, PATHOLOGY AND TREATMENT.

" ALL heavy horses are hogs." Heavy horses do not know when they have eaten enough. They have a craving for food, and if deprived of hay and grain, they will fill up upon any masticatory substance within their reach. They will even devour their dirty bedding. If not prevented, they will keep their stomachs constantly distended. They are all dyspeptics ; they are all flatulent. Heaves in horses corresponds to or is the same kind of disease in them that asthma is in man.

All asthmatic people are unhealthy feeders and over-eaters. They have a craving to keep the stomach full. If they cannot get the food which they most relish, they will eat what is set before them, or what they can get. They have no especially nice tastes or delicate appetites. They will fill up on the coarser aliments if they cannot obtain the finer. Food does not taste especially well to them, but they want to eat and will eat " to their fill." They are all dyspeptics of an especial type. They are all flatulent with carbonic acid gas. Their stomachs are full of fermenting products. These products are constantly being absorbed, the stomach being partially paralyzed and inactive. This special type of dyspepsia always develops a " gravelly diathesis," and a state of the system which renders the victim very susceptible to taking cold on the slightest exposure. The colds are more prone to affect the air passages than to take hold of other parts. This tendency to fasten upon the air passages arises from the fact that the alcoholic and acid products developed in the stomach by the yeast plants growing there, are largely eliminated through the air passages. This enervates, relaxes and partially paralyzes these parts, so that they become extremely susceptible to those causes productive of the states which we call "colds." These colds begin in the nasal passages and fauces, because these parts are the first and most directly exposed. A constant succession of these colds soon develops a chronic state of congestion in the parts, which we call catarrh.

All colds and catarrhs, when once started in the head (nasal passages and fauces), have a tendency to travel downward, towards the feet. An acute cold, like an eruptive fever, travels quickly; it only requires a few days to pass from the head to the feet. A chronic cold or catarrh travels slowly. This constant state of successive acute colds, or congestions, in the nose and fauces, when a gravelly diathesis is present, causes these parts to become especial seats of gravelly formations. As soon as this gravelly formation has firmly seated itself in the nasal cavities and fauces, we have established a confirmed type of gravelly catarrh, which — if the unhealthy feeding which generated it is kept up — will slowly work its way along down the air passages till it reaches the air cells, when asthmatic symptoms set in. It usually takes years, and sometimes many of them, for this gravelly disease or formation to reach the air cells. The rapidity of its progress is determined by the degree of indiscretions in eating, by habits of labor and exercise, and by the extent of exposures. As soon as this gravelly catarrh becomes established in the fauces and throat, small masses of a grayish, bluish, glutinous, jelly-like mucus are hawked out on rising and occasionally through the day. This glutinous mucus is tough and adhesive, like asthmatic mucus.

On microscopic examination it is found more or less filled with giant cells. (Figs. 5, 6, 7, 10, 12, 13, 17, 18, 19, 31 and 32, Plate XVI.) Many of these giant cells contain melanotic matter, and granules and small crystals of gravel. (Figs. 12, 13, 18, 19, 31 and 32, Plate XVI.)

As these giant cells break down, or are developed into filamentous mucus, the melanotic matter is spread out in streaks and little bands (Fig. 33, Plate XVI), or becomes diffused through the mass. Frequently crystalline fragments of considerable size are met with. (Figs. 20, 23, 24, 28, 29, Plate XVI; 39, 40, 41, 42, Plate XVII.) Every fresh cold aggravates this condition. If the diet becomes healthy and the system be kept in good order, the gravelly catarrh will soon disappear to the extent of giving no inconvenience. Any continuous series of indiscretions, however, gets the system in a chronic state of susceptibility to colds, on the slightest exposure, and the gravelly state of the parts soon appears and continues until after the indiscretions have ceased.

No amount of medical treatment will cure this catarrh if its causes be continued. Medical treatment may ease and palliate; it cannot cure. This is the reason why catarrhs are so seldom done away with entirely through remedial means. Remove their cause, however, and curative processes begin and go on until the parts become sound and normal in the course of a year or more.

The primary cause of asthma in all its forms is unhealthy and over-alimentation.

The secondary cause is the gravelly diathesis, which is gradually developed by long-continued, special, unhealthy and undue feeding.

The tertiary causes, or consequential factors are a series of colds, for which the system has become fitted through the operation of the primary cause.

The deranging effect of these causes determines the localization of excessive gravelly formation in the air passages.

Accessory to, and as a consequence of these causes, comes in the development of a species of Spirilina (*Spirilina Asthma — Salisbury.* Pl. XVII, Figs. 76, 77, 78, 79 and 80), forming long, very tough, adhesive ropes, which it is almost impossible to tear loose from their fastenings by coughing.

The more rapidly and prolifically this vegetation develops, the tougher and more adhesive the mucus, and the more terrible the paroxysms of difficult breathing and coughing.

These spiral plants, when wound around with tough mucous filaments, have a luminous appearance under the microscope, and can be readily made out.

The tougher the mucus and the harder the paroxysms, the more abundant will the *Spirilina Asthma* be found to be.

The exciting cause of the paroxysms may be anything that enervates or paralyzes the pulmonary nerves or that will (when inhaled and coming in contact with the diseased surfaces) produce enough disturbance to temporarily and sufficiently paralyze the parts and bring about the secretion of very tough, ropy, sticky mucus. This mucus fills the air cells and minute bronchiæ to such an extent that the inhaled air cannot get back of and behind the tough secretion, and enable the victim to expectorate it.

The inhaled material excitant of these paroxysms may be any one of a great variety of bodies. The malady groups itself into several well-marked forms, each form being determined by the special excitements, states and conditions of the system and its organs, and the substance which, when inhaled, arouses the paroxysm. In spasmodic asthma, the exciting cause of the paroxysm may be a full stomach of indigestible and fermenting food, and the absorption of carbonic acid gas during the night; the inhaling carbonic acid gas or any other irritating gases; vitiated air, dust, over-exertion, colds, etc., etc. In this form of the disease paroxysms may come at any time of the year or at any hour of the day, but are more prone to be troublesome during the latter part of the night on account of the absorption of carbonic acid gas from the stomach, which has been developed from the fermenting foods eaten during the day and gradually absorbed after retiring. The absorption of this gas by 2 o'clock or 3 o'clock a. m. has so paralyzed the nerves of the lungs that an asthmatic paroxysm comes on.

" Hay fever " comes on during the period of " haying," and is excited by the exhalations and spores emanating from fermenting and drying grass. There is a species of fucidium growing on the blades of fermenting and drying grass which often excites paroxysms.

In Rose asthma, or "rose cold," the odor of the rose excites the paroxysm. This may occur at any season of the year when inhaling the perfume of that flower.

"Malarial asthma" comes on in the middle and northern States from the 10th to the 25th of August, and marks, in the locality where it occurs, the beginning of the rapid development of malarial vegetation. This is a very common and aggravated form of the disease, and is commonly known as "hay fever," but really has no connection with the harvesting of hay. In hay fever, rose cold or asthma, and in malarial asthma, the seat of the discomfort and irritation is mostly in the eyes, nasal cavity, fauces, larynx and upper bronchiæ. Later on in these forms of disease — when the gravelly development has reached the air cells — spasmodic asthma supervenes and aggravates the sufferings.

XXXVI.

DRINKS, FOODS, EXERCISE, CLOTHING AND TREATMENT IN SPASMODIC ASTHMA.

THE drinks, food, exercise and clothing are the same as in any of the fibrous diseases. These are given under the head of Uterine Fibroids (Uterine Fibrosis). The more rigidly the diet is followed and the more carefully the stomach is cleaned, the more rapid the gain.

Medication should be in the direction of improving digestion and assimilation, so as to stop forming poisonous and paralyzing gases, to check the formation of gravel, and to eliminate that already formed.

In handling asthma, if we desire to cure the disease, the real causes must be removed. These are unhealthy alimentation and the established gravel of the lungs. The paroxysms are purely symptomatic, and are the outward manifestation of the diseased and sensitive state of the internal parts; the weakened state of the parts is simply the result of the underlying causes heretofore named. While it may at times be desirable to make a patient as comfortable as possible during a paroxysm by using anodynes, palliatives and other " covering up " remedies, yet if you have twelve or twenty-four hours to work in before a paroxysm comes on, in nine cases out of ten there will be no paroxysm to treat. Remember that the paroxysm is not the disease; it is only a symptom of the disease. The disease is really unhealthy alimentation and gravel of the lungs. The time to treat, the time to medicate, the time to wash out and to eat properly; the time to improve digestion, to stop the gravelly formation and to thin the toughened secretions, is between the paroxysms, when the patient is comfortable. If the heart be not too weak, the following tonic will be found very satisfactory :

R/ Fluid Extract Wild Cherry Bark . . . . ℥ii
" " Grindelia Robusta Comp. . . . ℥iiiss
" " Sundew . . . . . . ℥i
" " Water Fennel Seed . . . . ℥i
" " (Either) Coca or Cinchona Comp. . ℥ii
" " Licorice . . . . . . ℥ii
" " Aromatic . . . . . . ℥ss
English Iodide of Potassium . . . . ℥iss
Oil. Menth. Pip. : . . . . . . gtt. x
S. Take a teaspoonful in a little water before each meal and on retiring.

This acts upon all the eliminating glands and thins the secretions, so that the gravelly matters are more readily eliminated from the lungs.

R/ Pure scale Pepsin . . . . ℥i
Pancreatine . . . . ℥ss
Mix and rub well together.
S. Take ten grains after each meal in a little clear tea.

R/ Pil. Digitaline ₁/₁₀₀ gr. each XXX.
S. Take a pill on retiring.

Apply a good Belladonna plaster between the shoulders. If constipated, take an Aperient Pill, or a stronger one if necessary, on retiring, so as to get one movement daily.

This treatment, together with the rigid diet, should be kept up by the month and continued until there is a perfect cure, if it takes three years. There need be no paroxysms after the treatment begins.

In malarial and other forms of asthma, arising from inhaling special bodies and odors, the treatment should continue during the winter, or during the season when the patient is feeling well and free from the outward and distressing manifestation of the disease.

The diet and treatment are similar to that of spasmodic

Asthma, and should be persisted in till the membranes of the air passages are in a perfect state of health.

In treating the paroxysms of the so-called "Hay Fever" (Malarial Asthma) the "Compound Menthol Ointment or Ice" will be found an admirable remedy for relieving the sufferer. It should be applied inside the nostrils and fauces, and outside the nose. Relief is almost instantaneous. This application can be made as often as desired. It does not cure, but lessens the force of the distressing paroxysms, and makes the patient comfortable till the malarial season is over (when frost comes), when treatment for a complete cure can be pushed forward.

XXXVII.

GRAVEL OF THE AIR PASSAGES. MELANOTIC MATTER AND
GIANT CELLS IN THEIR RELATION TO ASTHMA.

As before stated, I believe that melanotic matter is never
formed in the lungs, except in cases of gravel of these organs.
The melanotic matter always accompanies the formation of
gravelly matter in the pulmonary tissues, and the gravel never
occurs without its melanotic accompaniment. The so-called
" giant cells " are necessary consequences of the formation in
the bronchial membranes of insoluble particles of unorganized
and sometimes of organic matter. These " giant cells " are a
provision of nature to carry insoluble matters out of the follicles and parent cells.

The giant-cell membranes form around the particles of melanotic and gravelly granules and serve as vehicles for transporting them out of the parent cells and follicles, and finally out
of the organism. In all the early stages of gravelly catarrh of
the air passages, the gravelly matter is either granular or in
small crystals and concretions, as represented at Figs. 33, 34,
14, 20, 27 and 36, Plate XVI; 44, Plate XVII.

As the disease increases in severity and duration, the gravelly masses become — many of them — much larger, as represented at Figs. 28, 29, 38, 23, 24, 35, 37, Plate XVI; 39, 40,
41 and 42, Plate XVII.

Often the concretions become attached in the mouths or
bodies of the follicles, and grow to the size of a hazelnut, and
sometimes larger, before the tissues surrounding them break
down and let them escape. Occasionally the particles of gravel
become so thickly massed and so adhere together throughout

the tissues of the trachea and bronchial tubes, that their walls become calcified and we have bony tracheæ and bronchi. I have numerous calcified masses or concretions of gravel that have been expectorated, which range from the size of a pinhead to that of a hickory-nut. In all cases they are concretions made up of tunics or successive layers, the one over the other, which a polished cross section always shows. At Figs. 44, 45, 46 and 47, Plate XVII, are fusiform crystals, which are often found in great numbers in certain forms of asthma. These crystals are scattered more or less thickly throughout the sputa. Figs. 1, 2, 3 and 4, Plate XVI, are ciliated epithelial cells that have been loosened by the bronchial irritation and severe cough, and which are often found, in variable extent, in the sputa. The greater the bronchial irritation, the greater the number of these cells in the expectoration.

Such cells are very unlike the Asthmatos Ciliaris, for which some investigators have mistaken them. Figs. 5, 6, 7, 10, 12, 13, 54, 26, 31, 32, 17, 18 and 19, Plate XVI, are all various appearances and forms of giant cells. Some of these are filled with albuminoid globules (Figs. 5, 6, 7 and 10, Plate XVI), while others contain melanotic matter and gravelly granules, mixed with and in the albuminoid globules, as seen at Figs. 12, 13, 18, 19, 31 and 32, Plate XVI.

Figs. 13 and 19, Plate XVI, represent two of the giant cells bursted, and the granules of gravel and melanotic matter escaping. Fig. 33 represents masses of melanotic and gravelly granules already escaped from the giant cells. Figs. 8, 9 and 11, Plate XVI, represent the albuminoid matter of the giant cells, after it has escaped from the cells and run together in globules and beaded tubes of various sizes. This albuminoid matter is always present in bronchial congestions and irritations, wherever the giant cells are developed. The greater the bronchial disturbance, the larger the number of giant cells, and the greater the amount of albuminoid matter present. Figs. 49, 50, 51, 52, 53, 57, 58, 59, 60, 61 and 62, Plate XVI, represent spores and filaments of Leptothrix developing in and out of the epithelia and mucous cells, and which are found abundantly in expectoration. Figs. 63, 64, 65 and 66, Plate XVII, are spores and filaments of algæ developing in the expectorated mucus, often abundantly. Figs. 68, 70, 71, 72 and 73, Plate XVII, are spores developing in mucous cells, and spores and filaments developing out of the cells and mucus.

This is the Anabaina irregularis. Figs. 84 and 85, Plate XVII, are spores and filaments of another species of Anabaina.

Figs. 86 and 87, Plate XVII, are the spores and filaments of a species of Saccharomycetes developing in the sputa. Figs. 56 and 57, Plate XVII, represent a species of Sarcina which sometimes occurs in the expectoration. Figs. 67 and 68 represent mucous cells developing; some containing spores and others empty of their normal contents.

All these vegetations, except the Spirulina asthma, — Figs. 76, 77, 78, 79 and 80, Plate XVII, — are developed in consequence of certain conditions and states in the epithelium and secretions, and do not act at all as causes, though their presence may aggravate the symptoms.

XXXVIII.

FATTY INFILTRATION AND FATTY METAMORPHOSIS IN ORGANS
AND TISSUES, WITH THEIR CAUSE AND THE MEANS OF
CURE.

An organ or tissue never becomes either infiltrated with or
metamorphosed into fat, while in a normal or healthy state.

This process is inaugurated by an inactive, enervated or partially paralyzed state of the part. When a part becomes so inactive, enervated or paralyzed that its normal nourishment is
not drawn or supplied to it fast enough to support the histological elements and keep them from disintegrating, fat then begins to be infiltrated as a preservative and to keep up the bulk
of the part as far as possible.

Amputate a man's foot through the instep and in a year's
time the unused and inactive muscles of the calf of the leg become white with infiltrated fat.

When the heart is much paralyzed by the constant and long-
maintained pressure of carbonic acid gas in the stomach, so that
its pulsations are weak and intermittent, and often below fifty
beats to the minute, this organ is too inactive to obtain its normal fibrinous nourishment, and fat begins to be infiltrated. If
this process goes on for some years without reaching a fatal
result, the organ may attain partial calcification, especially if
there be a gravelly diathesis in the organism.

If instead of remaining a long time on the stomach, the fermentative processes soon pass into the small and large intestines
without resulting first in constipation and secondly in diarrhœa,
and if the yeasty state of the bowels continues for an extended
period, the presence of gas in this locality partially paralyzes

the kidneys. This intercepts the normal nourishment of their glandular tissue, and in consequence fat begins to be infiltrated, that the epithelial cells may be preserved from disintegration and death. So long as the cells have sufficient vitality to perform their glandular functions, so long will this infiltration continue: it is at length terminated when the gland cells of the malpighian corpuscles and tubuli uriniferi become metamorphosed into fat. To all intents and purposes the cells are then dead and unable to perform their duty of secreting urine. This is the final stage of Bright's Disease, or the stage of fatty metamorphosis, and is of brief duration, as death from uræmia soon intervenes.

When the liver, spleen and mesenteric glands become semi-paralyzed from fermentative processes, or so inactive from injuries to the nerves of the parts (or by reason of any other cause), that their requisite nourishment is not brought to them, fatty infiltration is liable to set in. If the cause or causes are not now removed, this process moves along, step by step, to a fatal result.

If a gravelly diathesis be present in the system, these glands may become more or less calcified before death. Fatty depositions first begin and are subsequently followed by calcified depositions, both of which then go on in the blood-vessels and glandular surfaces and ducts of the parts.

When the brain is, through similar causes, partially paralyzed and enervated, undue mental effort, anxiety, care and worry will precipitate fatty infiltration and metamorphosis in that organ. Fermentative processes in the stomach and bowels are always, in large measure, the cause of brain paralysis. No person with healthy digestive organs could ever fall a victim to fatty disease of either organs or tissues, unless such organs or tissues had been deprived of their normal activity by injuries to the nerves that go to the parts, or deprived of some part necessary to their activity, or by some mechanical device preventive of normal action.

The great majority of cases of fatty infiltration and meta-morphosis, are caused by unhealthy alimentation. Location and pathological condition determine the first point of organic attack. A strong organ or tissue will resist invasion longer than will a weak one. All fatty diseases arising from unhealthy feeding, and hastened and aggravated by over-work and worry, are curable during the stage of fatty infiltration. Cure is effected by the suppression of cause or causes. The primary cause is unhealthy alimentation. An aggravating influence may be either care, anxiety or over-work. All of these rob the digestive organs of that vital energy needed to carry on digestion.

Carbonic acid gas and the sulphides of hydrogen and ammonium in the alimentary canal, are all gases emanating from and developed by fermentative vegetable and animal foods. In perfect health, these gases are not so developed. It is when saccharine and amylaceous foods are too largely eaten, accompanied by moderate or insufficient exercise, that alcoholic and acid fermentation set in and soon develop large quantities of carbonic acid gas in stomach and bowels. If the vegetable aliment should be highly nitrogenous, sulphides of hydrogen and ammonium may also be moderately developed in the large intestines.

When nitrogenous animal foods are eaten largely, and the digestive powers become impaired, these foods begin to ferment; great amounts of sulphides of hydrogen and ammonium are then evolved and distend the alimentary canal. If the stomach be unable to digest the meats eaten, they lie there fermenting and decaying, and we have the stomach filled first with ammoniacal vapors, and afterwards with the gaseous sulphides of hydrogen and ammonium.

These gases, when eructated, taste like rotten eggs. If the meats pass from the stomach before being digested, they are apt to ferment and decay in the large intestines, which become distended with the gaseous sulphides.

Of all the poisonous agents, none paralyze and deaden parts more effectually and readily — though painlessly — than carbonic acid gas and the sulphides of hydrogen and ammonium. When inhaled in concentrated form these gases cause death by paralysis almost instantaneously, without suffering. When, however, they fill the alimentary canal in the perfectly healthy state, they apparently do but little injury at first, as they are not readily taken up. But should the mucous surfaces become paralyzed from prolonged immersion in these gases, they (the gases) are then quite readily absorbed, and little by little paralytic states of organs and tissues supervene, which sooner or later may and often do result in fatal disease.

I will here introduce the Drinks, Foods, Bathing, Exercise, etc., which I have successfully employed in handling Bright's Disease, and which are well adapted in general to fatty diseases of any organ or tissue.

XXXIX.

THE DRINKS, FOOD, BATHS, EXERCISE AND CLOTHING IN BRIGHT'S DISEASE.

Drinks. — Drink from one half to one pint of hot water, one and a half hours before each meal and on retiring, drinking slowly. The reasons for taking this hot water, and the results effected by its use, will be found in a previous chapter upon the use of hot water in all diseases. It should be taken as there described, and long enough before each meal to allow it time to leave the stomach before the food enters. Drink a cup (eight ounces) of clear tea, coffee or beef tea (made of beef freed from fat and connective tissue), at each meal. When thirsty, between two hours after a meal, and one hour before the next, drink hot water, clear tea or beef tea freed from fat or gelatine. Take no other drinks of any kind. Should the hot water sicken the stomach, sprinkle in just enough salt to take away the flat taste.

Food. — Eat the muscle pulp of lean beef made into cakes and broiled. This pulp should be carefully prepared as described in the previous chapter on the foods suitable to consumption. For variety, use also the steak (broiled) which is cut through the centre of a round of lamb or mutton; broiled quail, broiled oysters, broiled grouse, broiled woodcock, broiled snipe, broiled partridge and broiled codfish. The whites of eggs may be taken raw, poached or soft boiled. Avoid all fats as far as possible, using only salt and pepper for seasoning. Mustard mixed up with hot water, lemon juice or Worcestershire and Halford sauces may be used on meats if desired. A little celery may be eaten at dinner if desired. All other foods, drinks and condiments not mentioned above should be strictly prohibited.

This rigid diet should be kept up until all traces of albumen and casts disappear from the urine. When these have ceased to show themselves for a couple of weeks, the patient may be allowed one part of bread, toast or boiled rice, *by bulk*, and *not* by weight, to eight or ten parts of the beef eaten by him at a meal.

When this new departure has been continued for four weeks without the appearance of albumen or casts in the urine, the bread, toast or boiled rice may be increased to one part, *by bulk*, to six parts of the meat, and a piece of butter the size of a hickory-nut may be allowed for seasoning. After continuing these proportions for four weeks, if still no signs of albumen or casts show themselves, the bread, toast or rice may be increased to one part to five of the meat, with a little increase of the butter. Continue these proportions for one month. If no albumen or casts then appear in the urine, increase the bread, toast or boiled rice to one part to four of the meat, and continue this for a month longer. If all is still going on well at the expiration of this time, give during the succeeding month one part of bread, toast or boiled rice, to three of the meat, with a slight increase of the butter. Continue these proportions for three months, and then, if no sign of the disease be visible, increase the bread, toast or boiled rice to one part, by bulk, to two of the meat. Cracked wheat may now be brought in as a change from the rice. After continuing this diet for a couple of months more, if all goes well and no signs of albumen or casts appear in the urine, milk may be taken warm from the cow, two hours after breakfast and dinner. The patient should go out to the cow and drink the milk as soon as it comes from the teat and still contains all its animal life and heat. Begin with half a pint and gradually increase till the patient is taking a pint at a time, twice daily.

When this system of alimentation has been continued for a couple of months, if the patient still continues to thrive and is advancing gradually towards health, a little fruit may be indulged in after dinner. This indulgence, however, like all those progressive ones heretofore named, must be carefully controlled, and the patient must not be allowed over one peach, apple, orange or bunch of grapes per day. Sugar and cream also may be very moderately used in tea and coffee. This system of diet should be followed out for many months, and if the signs of the disease do not recur, it may be continued, gradually extending the diet list. It will be well, however, as a general rule, to continue to take two parts, *by bulk*, of lean meat (broiled or roasted) to one of all other food. If at any time during the treatment, after the albumen and casts have disappeared from the urine, they begin again to show themselves as the diet becomes more liberal, the patient should at once come squarely down to a lean meat diet as he did at the start, and proceed cautiously as before. The patient will lose in weight during the early part of the treatment, but this need not excite anxiety, for after the first few weeks this loss will be checked, and a gradual gain will set in.

Meals. — The meals should be taken at regular intervals, and it is better to eat alone or with those living on the same diet. All temptations should, as far as possible, be removed from the patient. If three meals a day are not sufficient to satisfy hunger, he may be allowed a nice piece of broiled steak between breakfast and dinner, and between dinner and supper. These extra meals should be taken at fixed and regular intervals. If care be taken in following out this plan of diet, it will not be long before the system gets in good order, the digestion and assimilation will go on smoothly, and the patient will eat largely and with great relish. He will often assure you that no food is so nice as a good broiled steak, and he will surprise you by eating one to two pounds at a meal. Never eat on a tired stomach. Rest one hour before and after each meal; eat slowly and masticate all food well.

Baths. — Take a soap and hot-water bath twice weekly for cleanliness, after which rub with a coarse towel till the skin is red. Every night or day sponge all over with hot water, in which put a tablespoonful of aqua ammonia to the quart of water; rub in well, and afterwards wipe dry.

Exercise. — Drive daily in an easy vehicle as much as is possible without fatigue. If not able to walk or drive, the body and limbs should be rubbed, kneaded and pounded all over for from ten to twenty minutes — morning, noon and night — by some one who has the strength to do it thoroughly.

Clothing. — Wear flannel or silk next to the skin, and dress with comfortable warmth. On retiring, change all the clothing worn during the day, so that it may be thoroughly aired for the following morning. Keep the clothing sweet and clean by changing every second or third day.

The bed should be thrown open on rising, the bedding well aired during the day, and the bed not made up till the patient wishes to retire. Good ventilation is very essential. No tonics, mineral waters or external applications should be used: the physician will give such remedies as may be needed.

General Remarks. — Remember that the medicines cure nothing; they simply assist in keeping the machine in good running order, while the cure is effected by rigid alimentation — an alimentation freed as far as possible from all paralyzing and fat-forming elements. The constant and long-continued fermentation of vegetable food, fruits and sweets in the stomach and bowels keeps the digestive organs all the time filled with carbonic acid gas. After a time this gas so paralyzes the cells of those surfaces with which it comes in contact, that they lose their normal selective power and begin to take up, little by little, increasing amounts of carbonic acid gas, yeast, vinegar, etc., which are carried into the circulation, and thus reach every part of the organism.

The heart, liver, lungs, kidneys, spleen and brain are among the first organs to suffer. The organs that are the first and most liable to be paralyzed are the kidneys and heart; the portal glands are the next. It is not sufficient to search for the cause of disease in weekly and monthly exposures, but those of daily and hourly occurrence must be considered. The either healthy or pathological acts which create healthy or diseased habits must be regular, frequent and long continued, before they can become states of health or established conditions of disease. We must reach the underlying causes before we can cure. We may relieve and seemingly cure without knowing or removing causes, but such relieving and curing is not permanent. We should remember that we bring about all these states and conditions by something which we daily and persistently do. This wrong-doing must cease; we may then advantageously employ any means that will help to gradually restore and establish healthy states and habits in the diseased structures.

XL.

THE DRINKS, FOOD, BATHS, EXERCISE AND CLOTHING IN DIABETES MELLITUS.

Drinks. — Drink hot water daily, as prescribed in previous chapters. Take also one half pint of beef tea — made from pure lean meat fibre, free from tendons, cartilage and fat — at each meal, and the same amount between two hours after breakfast and one hour before dinner ; between two hours after dinner and one hour after supper, and between two hours after supper and one hour before breakfast the next morning — making in all, three pints of beef tea in the twenty-four hours. Take no other drinks of any kind or description, unless it be a few mouthfuls of clear weak tea or coffee with the medicine.

Food. — Eat the muscle pulp of lean beef, carefully prepared according to the process described in the previous chapter on food in consumption. When cooked, put it on a hot plate, and season to taste with butter, pepper and salt. Either Worcestershire, Halford or Chutney sauce may be used on meats if desired. A little celery may be eaten at each meal. The urine should flow at the rate of three pints daily, and stand at or near a density of 1.020. This state of things should be continuously present for five or six weeks before bread and vegetable food are ventured upon. When it is thought that the proper time has arrived, begin by allowing the patient one mouthful of bread at each meal. Take this bread after the meat is eaten. If after a few days the urine continues to remain at 1.010 density or thereabouts, and flows at the rate of three pints only in twenty-four hours, increase the bread to two mouthfuls at each meal. In this way make gradual and cautious advances, step by step, till at the end of four or five more weeks, the patient is taking two parts of lean meat to one of bread, toast, boiled rice, cracked wheat or potato. Keep up this kind of diet, in the above proportions, continuously for six consecutive months, before trying any fruits, except the lemon. A little lemon juice on the meats or after meals, may be indulged in at any time during the progress of the cure. After the patient is sufficiently recovered to take with safety one part of bread, toast, boiled rice or potato, to two of the meat, half a pint of clear tea or coffee may be substituted for the beef-tea at each meal. During the entire treatment all foods, drinks or condiments not herein named, should be rigidly avoided.

Baths. — Take a soap and hot-water bath twice weekly, for cleanliness, after which oil all over with sweet oil and glycerine, rubbing in well. Every night or day sponge all over with hot water, in which put from half to one ounce of aqua ammonia to the quart of water; rub in well and wipe dry afterward. Every day put a teaspoonful of diluted nitro-muriatic acid in six ounces of hot water, and rub in thoroughly over the region of the liver. Keep this up until a miliary eruption appears, when stop it till the eruption disappears; then resume it until eruption again shows itself, and so on during the progress of cure.

Clothing. —Wear flannel or silk next the skin and dress with comfortable warmth. On retiring, change all clothing worn during the day, so that it may be thoroughly aired for the following morning. Keep the clothing sweet and clean by changing every other day. The bed should be thrown open on rising, and the bedding well aired during the day, and the bed not made till it is time to retire.

Exercise. — Drive and walk daily in the open air, as much as is possible without fatigue. Four to six hours in the twenty-four should be spent in this way. If not able to walk or drive, the body and limbs should be rubbed and pounded all over for twenty minutes, morning, noon and night, by some one who has the strength to do it thoroughly.

Meals. — The meals should be taken at regular intervals, and it is better not to sit down at a table where others are indulging in all kinds of food. Eat alone or only with those who are on the same kind of diet. After the system gets into good running order, which is indicated by the urine flowing at the rate of from three to four pints daily, and standing at a density of from 1.020 to 1.026, the appetite becomes good and often ravenous. Frequently in this stage of the cure more than three meals a day are desired. This wish should be gratified by allowing the patient a nice broiled steak between breakfast and dinner, and between dinner and supper. These extra meals should be taken at fixed and regular hours every day.

General Remarks. — Avoid all anodynes and other medicinal agents which tend to get the stomach, bowels, kidneys and skin out of order. The cure is accomplished by removing the unhealthy alimentation that has culminated in the disease, and in furthering the removal of the pathological states of the deranged organs, by the use of such remedial agents as assist in restoring normal, healthy action.

By judiciously and persistently following out the foregoing plan of alimentation, treatment, etc., the diseased organs and system generally soon begin to take on a more healthy state.

The urine contains every succeeding day a smaller proportion of sugar; its density lessens steadily, its quantity decreases, the color heightens, the appetite improves, the eyes grow brighter and brighter, the skin gradually loses its dryness and becomes more soft and oily, and the mucous membranes less and less feverish and dry; the thirst ceases, and the entire organism takes on, little by little, yet certainly and surely, the actual appearances, states and conditions of health.

In less than one week's time after this treatment is thoroughly entered upon, the quantity of urine decreases from gallons to about two quarts per diem; the density falls from 1.040 to 1.060, down to 1.026 to 1.034, varying with the advancement and severity of the disease. The thirst usually ceases in about three days, after which the sufferings of the patient are comparatively slight.

The least deviation on the part of the patient from the course marked out can be at once detected by the watchful and expert physician. A single mouthful of bread, vegetables, fruit, sauce, sugar or any fermenting farinaceous or saccharine food will elevate the density of the urine many degrees, by increasing the sugar in it, and the quantity voided will be much greater. The physician should be able to perceive immediately any departure of the patient, and call him to strict account. No one need hope to handle this disease successfully, without an unfaltering observance of the foregoing rules and regulations.

Medicines alone will not cure the disease. They are merely aids to the restoration of healthy states, after the cause, or the unhealthy alimentation is removed. None but reckless feeders ever have this disease unless, as occurs in rare instances, it has been imperfectly developed by local injuries. As the desires and appetites of the patient have to be wholly repressed and ignored, the physician must endeavor to inspire him with such faith and earnestness that his soul and body may make a firm stand against the awful cravings of diseased organs. His only hope lies in the maintenance of an unwavering determination to carry on the good work; otherwise he will so often yield to the morbid longings for fermentable food, as to render his cure impossible. The patient can tear down more in one minute, by indulging in the forbidden, than the physician can build up in three days. Hence the odds are with the downward course of the patient, unless the physician can instill into him such a sense of duty and responsibility to himself and to others, that the will to do rightly under all circumstances will conquer the intensity of perverted appetites. Organic diseases arising from defective or unhealthy alimentation are the result of confirmed habits in eating too exclusively and too continuously such food as cannot be well digested in the way and proportion in which it is taken, and is unfitted for assimilation. The chemical and vital changes of fermentation, decay and cryptogamic development set in, resulting in the production of agents debilitating and poisonous to the various vital organs which they reach through their being more or less taken up by the gland cells of the digestive apparatus. Such desires become fixed pathological habits in the organ or organs affected, and have been brought on by such organs being continuously compelled to do and to be exposed to labors which they are unfitted to perform and endure, without becoming over-taxed, enervated, deranged, paralyzed and changed in function, and eventually in structure.

To produce these states, conditions and changes requires time and unvarying exposure to the before-mentioned abnormal causes and labors. To cure them, also requires time and a persistent long-continued avoidance of all productive causes, as well as the constant and unflinching use of such food and medical means as will keep the system in undeviatingly perfect running order. Success in this direction will be indicated by the urine flowing at the rate of about three pints daily, standing at a density of 1.020, clear, no sediment being deposited on cooling, and no sugar, albumen, or other pathological body or condition being present; the bowels moving once or twice a day, and at the regular time; no pains or aches; head clear, no dizziness; skin and mucous membranes in good order; mind cheerful, and all the normal functions going on in a healthy manner.

In this disease, the lobules of the liver — or that portion of the gland which is connected directly with the blood-vessels, and which organizes glycogenic matter or animal sugar — is the part which is directly involved. This portion of the liver is over-active, and makes more animal sugar than is required. The excess of sugar has to be eliminated, and this additional stress of work is thrown upon the kidneys. Soon they too become over-active, and little by little are indirectly involved in the disease. To effect a cure, we must cut off (as far as possible) all food which goes to make animal sugar. This includes vegetable food, animal fats, tendon and connective or glue tissues and cartilage. Also all excess in drinks. Abstinence in these respects will lessen the labor of the diseased parts and by degrees subdue their excessive activity. Normal states then ensue, and if these are well established for a few months, and accompanied by appropriate medication, they break up the diseased habit and restore normal conditions, which, becoming in their turn permanent, finally and thoroughly cure the disease.

XLI.

REMARKABLE RESEMBLANCE BETWEEN THE SYMPTOMS AND IN-
TERCURRENT, ABNORMAL CONDITIONS OF DIABETES AND
THOSE OF CHRONIC DIARRHŒA.

THERE is a remarkable similarity between the complications and many of the symptoms and tendencies of chronic diarrhœa and those of diabetes. . In both diseases there is a highly saccharine or glycogenic condition of the system, and a peculiar abnormal tendency to fermentative changes. In both there is a marked tendency to heart disease ('Thrombosis of Virchow) and tuberculosis, with paralytic tendencies and maladies of the eye and ear. In the one disease there is a highly saccharine condition of the feces and alimentary secretions, and in the other, of the urine. In the former, the liquids of the body are flowing off through the bowels, and in the latter through the urinary organs. Yeast plants are developed largely in the increased excretions of each disease.

In chronic diarrhœa the urine is scanty : in diabetes, the bowels are constipated. In both diseases there are marked dyspeptic symptoms with sour eructations. The mouth and fauces are either dry or watery ; tongue clean and red ; marked thirst and appetite, and a constantly increasing emaciation, with inability to maintain the temperature of the body up to the normal temperature : from this inability, creeping, chilly sensations result.

XLII.

DRINKS, FOOD, EXERCISE, BATHING AND TREATMENT IN UTE-
RINE FIBROIDS AND IN OTHER FIBROUS GROWTHS AND THICK-
ENINGS, IN LOCOMOTOR ATAXY AND ALL SCLEROTIC STATES:
IN OVARIAN TUMORS, GOITRE AND ALL EXCESSIVE DEVELOP-
MENTS OF CONNECTIVE OR GLUE TISSUE OCCURRING IN PARTS
TO WHICH THEY DO NOT NORMALLY BELONG.

THE scope of this work not admitting of an exhaustive description of the pathological conditions and processes of the
above-named diseases, I shall do no more than state that all
these fibrous growths and thickenings, and all excessive developments in connective tissue, where such development does not
normally belong, are the outcome of unhealthy alimentation.

When vegetables, sweets and fruits have been too exclusively
and continuously used, and when they ferment in the stomach,
as heretofore described, this fermentation, both alcoholic and
acid, gradually increases until quantities of carbonic acid gas and
plants belonging to the genera Saccharomyces and Mycoderma
(with the products, beer and acid) are largely developed, especially in persons of sedentary habits. When these products have
saturated the intestinal track and paralyzed the cells of the villi
and follicles so that digestion is impaired, the cells of the villi
suspend their normal selective power, and instead of taking up
nutritious products only, they take up the poisonous and paralyzing products of fermentation indiscriminately, and transmit them
into the circulation. Whenever an organ or tissue lies near the
seat of the development and accumulation of these products of
fermentation, that organ or tissue becomes in turn partially paralyzed. The blood-vessels then dilate, and a stasis in the blood
stream of the parts is established, so that nutritious products

nourish such semi-paralyzed tissues exclusively, and there is hypernutrition of the parts under a state of partial death. Hence the growth is painless and not inflammatory. All painless growths come under this head.

This class of abnormal developments are poorly supplied with nerves and blood-vessels, and are hence destined to have a brief existence only.

It will be seen that there are three factors to be considered in such developments: —

1. Too exclusive feeding upon one class of foods, which are generally those fermenting readily with alcoholic and acid yeasts.

2. The paralyzing influence of the products of the fermentation of the foods eaten.

3. The excessive nourishment of the connective and other tissues in which the growths may occur.

In the cure of such growths these factors are to be eliminated. The following treatment is productive of the best results in this direction.

Drinks. — Drink a pint of hot water one to two hours before each meal, and half an hour before retiring. From fifteen to thirty minutes should be taken for drinking this water, so that the stomach may not be uncomfortably distended. The objects and uses of this hot water are fully described in an earlier chapter, which should be carefully read. When thirsty, between two hours after a meal and one hour before the next, drink hot water, clear tea or crust coffee. Take no other drinks of any kind at any time. At meals drink one cup (eight ounces) of clear tea.

Food. — Eat the muscle pulp of lean beef, prepared as described in the chapter on " Food in Consumption." Either Worcestershire, Halford or Chutney sauce may be used on meats if desired. A little celery may be eaten at each meal. Avoid all other food, drinks and condiments. This rigid diet should be kept up until the fibrous growths have either mostly or entirely disappeared, when bread, toast, boiled rice and cracked wheat may be gradually brought into the diet list. Begin then to take other meats, such as lamb, mutton, game, fish and whole steaks. If the fibrous growths begin to increase at any time, come squarely and immediately down to the muscle pulp of beef, and continue it until all traces of the growth have disappeared. Then begin as before to bring other foods gradually into use, moving along watchfully and carefully, keeping the stomach clean, the urine clear, and standing at 1.015, and the appetite good. It takes from one to three years of determined work to remove fibrous diseases thoroughly, and to break up all the diseased appetites, cravings and desires that have been at the bottom of the conspiracy in producing such grave pathological states.

For the first few months the patient will lose in weight from the loss of fat and connective tissue. This, however, is a favorable indication, and need excite no uneasiness. After a while, the increase in blood, muscle, bone and nerve will be greater than the shrinkage, when a gain in weight will take place. This gain will be slow, but it will be all the time steadily advancing in the direction of the healthy state.

The physician and patient must both be satisfied with this steady improvement, even if it should be quite slow. It is the only way open to a perfect cure and to perfect health. Extirpating a growth never removes the cause, and never results in a radical cure. The same old alimentation may develop still other and further growths. I have now several cases in hand where operations were performed but a few years ago, and already fibrous tumors weighing from twelve to thirty pounds have appeared.

Meals. — The meals should be taken at regular intervals. It is better to eat alone, or only with those who are living on the same diet. All temptations should, as far as possible, be removed from the patient.

If three meals a day are not sufficient to satisfy hunger, the patient may be allowed a nice piece of broiled steak between breakfast and dinner, and dinner and supper. These extra meals should be taken at fixed and regular intervals. If care be taken in following out this plan of diet, it will not be long before the system gets into good order; the digestion and assimilation will go on nicely, while the patient will eat largely and with great relish. The appetite becomes so good and the relish for the beef is so great that you need not be surprised to see from one to two pounds eaten at each meal. The patient should be cautioned never to eat when fatigued, and to rest before meals as well as after. The food should be eaten slowly and well masticated.

Baths. — Take a soap and hot-water bath twice a week for cleanliness, after which oil all over with glycerine and water, and rub well from the head towards the feet. Every night or day, sponge all over with hot water, into which put two or four teaspoonfuls of aqua ammonia to the quart of water; rub in well and wipe dry.

Exercise. — Drive daily as much as possible without fatigue. If not able to walk or drive, the body and limbs should be rubbed well from the head towards the feet, for ten to twenty minutes, morning, noon and night, by some one who has the strength to do it passively, thoroughly and well, without exciting the patient.

Clothing. — Wear flannel or silk next the skin and dress with comfortable warmth. On retiring, change all clothing worn during the day, so that it may be thoroughly aired for the following morning. Keep the clothing sweet and clean by changing often. The bed should be thrown open on rising, and the bedding well aired during the day, the bed not being made up until the patient wishes to retire. Good ventilation is very essential at all times.

Medical Treatment. — Remember that the medicines cure nothing; they simply aid in keeping the machine in good running order, while rigid and careful alimentation is effecting the

cure, — an alimentation freed as much as possible from all elements which tend to form connective tissue, or to paralyze the
parts.

Tincture of iodine and iodoform may often be brought in
advantageously for local applications. The iodides and bro-
mides of potassium, ammonium and sodium may at times be
used internally to stimulate the digestive organs. Pepsin and
pancreatine taken during or after meals may, under the proper
conditions, help in so far as they promote digestion and assimilation. The great aim should be to keep all parts of the system
in the most perfect running order possible.

XLIII.

FIBRÆMIA OR HÆMAFIBROSIS.

THIS is the excessive development of glue or connective tissue — in skeins — in the blood-vessels and the blood stream.

These skeins, when found in this locality, indicate approaching danger in the shape of thrombosis, embolism and paralysis. They say to us that the glue tissue is badly and abnormally fed, so much so, that it begins to develop in skeins in the blood stream, where it does not properly belong.

(See Plate VI, Figs. 1 and 2, and Plate VII, Figs. 1, 2, 3 and 4. There is danger of fibrous growths and thickenings in the blood apparatus, taking the shape of thrombi and thickenings of the valves and walls of the heart and blood-vessels.)

This condition conduces to more or less disturbance in the action of the heart. The pulsations are usually slower and weaker than is normal, with more or less interruptions. The head is often muddy or somewhat mixed, and at times confused, with occasional spells of dizziness. Prickling sensations are present in the extremities to a greater or lesser extent : there is a general feeling of lassitude, and an inability and indisposition to all exertion, whether mental or physical. Wakefulness, anxiety and nervousness are frequent accompaniments of this state. If the cause — which is unhealthy alimentation — is not removed, the course of the disease progresses, and the patient is sooner or later prostrated with paralysis caused by thrombosis and embolism.

The diet, drinks and treatment in this disease are the same or similar to those adopted in treating uterine fibroids and fibrous growths generally in any part of the body, and are as follows : —

Drinks. — Drink one pint of hot water from one to two hours before each meal, and before retiring, in the method and for the objects advanced in a previous chapter upon the use of hot water. Drink a cup of clear tea or coffee at each meal. When thirst is felt between two hours after a meal and one hour before the next, drink hot water or hot clear tea, made weak and without sugar. Take no other drinks of any kind. If the hot water should sicken the stomach, either squeeze in a little lemon juice, put in a little clear tea or sprinkle in a little salt.

Food. — Eat the muscle pulp of beef prepared as described in the chapter on food in consumption. The cakes should be quite well cooked, placed on a hot plate and nicely seasoned with butter, pepper and salt. Mustard mixed with hot water, lemon juice, Worcestershire or Halford sauces may be used in moderation if desired. All other foods, drinks and condiments should be avoided till the skeins of connective tissue have entirely disappeared from the blood, and the normal action of the heart is restored. Then gradually bring in the bread foods and other lean meats, with a moderate quantity of vegetables.

Medicines. — The medicines to be used are simply such as are necessary to aid digestion and assimilation, and to keep the bowels open once a day.

Baths. — Take a soap and hot-water bath about twice a week, after which rub well and wipe dry. Every night or day, sponge all over with hot water, in which put two or three teaspoonfuls of aqua ammonia to the quart. Use a little soap with the sponge bath.

Exercise. — Exercise should be taken either by driving or by being rubbed. Never exercise to fatigue.

Plate VI, Fig. 1, shows the skeins in the blood of a patient in this condition, before any absolute paralysis has taken place, though for some time previous he had a slow, weak, intermittent pulse, standing at from 48 to 54 per minute, and the interruptions from 8 to 12 per minute. Head mixed, confused and unable to attend to business. Very nervous and wakeful nights. Dreams troubled and always tired and languid. Prickling, numb feelings in extremities, with coldness of feet and hands.

Plate VI, Fig. 2, represents the skeins of connective tissue in the blood of a lady patient eighty-five years of age. She has had a most remarkable constitution; has always been in comparatively good health as long as she could be active. During several years previous to this examination, she had lived chiefly on bread foods and tea, on account of loss of teeth. At the time of the examination she was very dizzy and confused, and liable to fall at any time when on her feet : ideas somewhat mixed ; prickly sensations in extremities and heart-beats slow and intermittent.

Plate VII, Figs. 1, 2, 3 and 4, represent skeins of connective tissue in the blood of a man of most remarkable constitution, a possessor of large wealth, who had always fed extravagantly upon all the "good things" that money could buy, and excellent cooks could prepare. For three years previous to my seeing him, he had been given up to die, and had already been tapped 79 times during that period. All the glands of the abdominal cavity were enlarged and hardened, and the abdomen largely distended. The skin was jaundiced ; eyes glassy ; feet and extremities cold and often painful and dropsical. The pulse ranged from 44 to 50 with at least 25 interruptions to the minute. Head mixed and bewildered, and body and mind weak and incapacitated from acting with any directness of purpose.

XLIV.

FATTY INFILTRATION AND FATTY METAMORPHOSIS OF THE FAS-
CICULI OF THE VOLUNTARY AND INVOLUNTARY MUSCULAR
TISSUE.

THIS very common disease is usually the outcome of long
continued, unhealthy feeding, which has impaired digestion and
assimilation by slow but sure degrees. The culminating point
in this process of degeneration is reached when the digestive
organs become a well-established apparatus for the development
of the various alcoholic and acid yeasts, as well as the yeasts,
which produce fermentation and decay in the various animal
foods. The entire system now begins to suffer from an insuffi-
ciency of normal nourishment, and from the poisonous proper-
ties of the different products of various fermentations. These
products are taken up and gradually saturate, enervate, poison
and paralyze the whole organism.

Other things being equal, the more inactive the person, the
more rapidly these deranged conditions advance. As soon as
the muscular tissue in any part becomes so enervated and paralyzed that there is danger of death and disintegration of the
weaker fasciculi, fat is infiltrated into them, to preserve them
from decay. This cautious process well displays the wisdom
delegated to our machines, to afford us time for repentance,
reform and repair, if we have the knowledge and disposition
thereunto. If we are without the knowledge, or have the
knowledge and not the disposition, the abnormal fatty changes
continue their gradual invasion of the muscular fasciculi, both
voluntary and involuntary. The patient grows more and more
enervated, more and more bloodless, till the parent fibrin cells of
the arterial extremities in the blood glands become involved, so

that blood is no longer organized, and death soon ensues from absolute starvation, as in the so-called *Pernicious Anæmia.*

If, however, we have the knowledge and disposition to reform and to remove these causes, and we go into the good work with our whole hearts, eating and drinking as we should, repair — even to perfect health — becomes a certainty.

This disease is always attended with muscular weakness — a want of muscular endurance. This increases as the malady advances, till its victims have to be supported in walking and finally become so weak that they are unable to turn in bed or to feed themselves. Such persons usually have a good and even ravenous appetite to the very last. In the final stage of the disease the body becomes greatly emaciated; eyes sunken and glassy; skin dry and wrinkled and voice husky. Death usually comes without pain, and they often die while endeavoring to satisfy the cravings of a starving body.

Fortunately, in a large majority of such cases, the diet is sufficiently conservative to preserve a very large percentage of the muscular fasciculi from being infiltrated with fat, so that life may be prolonged for many years and occasionally to advanced age.

The victim, however, is always more or less weak and unable to endure much exertion without some degree of prostration, from which he takes a long time to recuperate. A great number of people suffer more or less with this disease : in the majority however, it advances just far enough to make any considerable exertion more or less enervating.

In the lighter cases, less than one per cent of the fasciculi are fatty : in those a little further advanced two per cent is the rule : those still further advanced have three, four and five per cent, and in others from five per cent upwards of the fasciculi are fatty. When the disease affects above five to ten per cent of the fasciculi, it produces marked weakness.

When the physician has doubts regarding the character of the disease, a few muscular fasciculi may be snatched out instantly from the weaker muscles by means of a small barbed instrument with a spring. It is done so quickly that scarcely any pain is experienced. A few specimens taken out and examined microscopically will soon settle the question beyond all doubt.

As soon as a positive diagnosis is reached, and you find this disease to be present, the blood, urine and feces are to be carefully examined, that you may know what food is not digested, what food is fermenting and decaying, and to get at the condition of the glands, etc. All food which the digestive organs are unable to assimilate should at once be stopped. The stomach and bowels should be carefully washed out with hot water, one and a half hours before each meal, and only such food should be allowed as can be best digested. Usually this will be nothing but the muscle pulp of beef. Only about four to six ounces of clear tea or hot water should be allowed as a drink towards the close of each meal. All exercise should be passive. The patient should rest an hour before and after each meal and avoid all mental worries and excitements. In short, the same course of treatment in general should be adopted as is used in Bright's and in other fatty diseases.

XLV.

SOME OF THE DISEASES PRODUCED BY TOO EXCLUSIVE FEEDING
UPON AMYLACEOUS AND SACCHARINE FOODS AND FRUITS,
WITH THE DIET TO BE USED FOR THEIR CURE.

Vegetable Dyspepsia, or the first Stage of Consumption.

This arises from the too exclusive and long-continued use of
vegetable or amylaceous and saccharine foods and fruits, or
either of them.

The stomach is the first organ to suffer. In man this organ
is mainly designed for digesting lean meats. It may be called
a purely carnivorous organ. It requires lean meats to excite a
normal quantity of healthy secretions in its glandular follicles
for digestion, and the healthy excitation of these secretions
stimulates the muscular fibres to maintain those normal downward peristaltic movements which are necessary for physiological digestion and transmission.

The stomach does not digest amylaceous and saccharine
foods, fruits and fats. These are digested by the secretions
that are poured out into the duodenum by the liver, pancreas,
and glands of Lieberkuhn and Bruner.

Hence the too exclusive and long-continued use of vegetable,
and especially amylaceous and saccharine food, fills the stomach
with materials which do not stimulate it even enough to pass
them along to where they are digested, in consequence of which
they lie so long in this organ that fermentative processes supervene little by little, and we have the stomach filled with carbonic acid gas, sugar, alcohol, acid and alcoholic and acid yeast
plants. These products of fermentation soon begin to paralyze
the follicles and muscular walls of the stomach, so that it becomes

flabby and baggy, and will hold an unusual amount of trashy foods and fluids. The organ has been turned into a veritable sour " yeast pot," and we have the first stage of the disease known as vegetable dyspepsia of the stomach, or the first stage of consumption.

In this stage of the disease, the stomach is almost constantly distended with gas, which is only partially relieved by the frequent sour eructations.

Yeast plants are rapidly developed in the organ, and every particle of vegetable food which is taken in immediately begins to ferment, — the stomach being converted into an apparatus for manufacturing beer, alcohol, vinegar and carbonic acid gas. This carbonic acid gas soon begins to paralyze the gastric nerves, and the follicles of the mucous membranes of the organ commence to pour out a stringy viscid mucus, in considerable quantities. This, together with the partial paralysis, produces a relaxed, dilated state of the blood-vessels, so that a congestion (with a low state of vitality) results. The epithelial surfaces and connective tissue layer beneath them, then begin to increase in thickness, and if this process and state continue long enough, we have a gastric fibroid which may terminate in scirrhus of the organ. If, however, the person is fairly active, so as to shake the food out of the stomach into the duodenum and small bowels, or if the pyloric valve becomes sufficiently paralyzed to remain open, so that the food and liquids flow into the small bowels soon after being swallowed, then danger of gastric thickening is lessened : the patient feels much more comfortable and thinks he is greatly improved. The disease, however, is no better. It has simply changed its base of action and is transferred from the stomach to the small bowels. This is the second and most dangerous stage, being vegetable dyspepsia of the small bowels.

The exercise, habits of living, eating and drinking may be such as to detain the disease in this stage a long while. There is then great danger of the passage of Mycoderma spores (and the products developed by their multiplication) into the blood stream. Should this occur, we are in the second or transmissive stage of Consumption. In this stage of the disease, the bowels are more or less constipated. Generally speaking, the more constipated they are, the greater the danger.

An inactive, sedentary life, and a great disturbance of the bowels with carbonic acid gas and other yeasty products, may early paralyze the ileo-cæcal valve so far as to let the fermenting products pass readily and freely into the large bowels. The danger of having the yeast spores transmitted is then lessened by the free passage of the spores into the colon, where they go on exciting fermentation in the various fermenting foods used. This soon results in many copious, yeasty evacuations during the night or early every morning and forenoon. Sometimes there are twenty or more passages daily. The passages are light and bulky, and have but little weight. They are sour yeast. This is the third stage of Vegetable Dyspepsia or Chronic Diarrhœa, or more strictly speaking, Consumption of the Bowels. The disease, if left to itself, and if the foods producing it are kept up, may run on for months or even years. I have treated and cured cases that had been running on for from fifteen to twenty years.

In all cases of this stage of the disease, the large bowel becomes greatly thickened, and often in severe cases is almost entirely closed up. This thickening goes on quite rapidly in the connective tissue layer, and in the epithelial lining of the bowel. The folds of the bowel soon become greatly enlarged and are elongated from a few inches to a foot or more extra in length.

If the patient lives long enough, and is on a curative diet, these folds and the thickening gradually disappear by absorption, though sometimes the elongated folds slough away partially decayed. Occasionally, in severe cases, from three to four years are required to remove all traces of the disease and all thickenings of the bowel. As long as the thickenings are present, there will be more or less of a thick, jelly-like, ropy, viscid mucus, coming away every day or every few days or weeks, according to the condition and severity of the disease.

In consumption of the bowels, the lungs almost invariably become involved before death. Checking the diarrhœa with astringents — while the fermenting foods are kept up — only aggravates the disease in the end and endangers lung invasion.

Summer Complaint in Children.

The summer diarrhœas in children are of the same character as the so-called Chronic Diarrhœa, previously described. It is essentially a disease of unhealthy or defective feeding, and readily yields to the simplest treatment, by removing the cause and substituting food that will not ferment with yeast.

As soon as green vegetables and fruit begin to appear in early summer, children live almost entirely upon this kind of food at the expense of more substantial aliments.

The same symptoms and pathological lesions, in the same order, result as has been previously described under the head of chronic diarrhœa, and the disease yields readily to the same treatment.

Influence of Army Diet in Producing Diseases of Soldiers.

In the army there is in all the men a peculiar chronic condition of the alimentary membranes, excited by frequent fermentation of amylaceous matters too long retained, and which condition does not run on to chronic diarrhœa unless some enervating cause — such as over-fatigue, dysentery, typhoid, bilious, remittent or intermittent fever, or other cause — debilitates the system, and further impairs the condition of the alimentary membranes. This is evidenced by the almost universal condition of the alimentary canal in apparently healthy soldiers who are shot dead in battle. (See Eng. Surg. and Med. Hist. of Crimean War.)

The follicles of the large intestines are more or less enlarged and frequently disintegrated, leaving ulcers. The amylaceous, army biscuit diet of the common soldiers, besides its fermentative and carbonic acid poisoning effects, does not furnish to the system the proper proportion of ingredients for healthy alimentation and nutrition. Hence a scorbutic condition results, which renders the disease an obstinate one to treat, unless this state is recognized and particularly attended to. This explains the reasons why the vegetable acids, combined with potassa and iron, are so useful in treating this disease. Rochelle salts are admirably adapted for exciting intestinal epithelial activity, and secretion and absorption in the alimentary canal.

Any one kind of food too long continued has a tendency to produce systemic derangements of a scorbutic type. Amylaceous matters, too exclusively used, tend to excite abnormal actions in the parent epithelial cells of the mucous surfaces and of the glands; while any one kind of animal food, too long and too exclusively eaten, produces derangements which show themselves more strongly in skin and mouth. A too free use of oils and fatty food, and of alcoholic beverages, produces the red, blotched face, and swollen carbunculated nose, oily surface, and erythematous swelling and redness of the skin generally.

Salt meats produce a dry, scaly eruption upon the surface, with spongy, swollen and discolored gums; loosened teeth, and a watery, flabby, often bloody tongue; pains in the limbs and back resembling those of chronic rheumatism; leaden-hued features; offensive breath; patches of extravasated blood in various parts of the body; hard, contracted condition of the muscles; stiffness of the joints; diarrhœa and hemorrhage from mucous surfaces generally; mental depression and indisposition to any kind of exertion. From this scorbutic condition — produced in all the men by the want of the necessary variety in their food — arises a long train of the most fatal and most obstinate diseases of the army. Among these may be mentioned chronic diarrhœa; the so-called muscular rheumatism; dysentery; hospital gangrene in wounds; tuberculosis; fibrinous depositions in the heart; the clogging up of pulmonary vessels with fibrinous clots; paralytic conditions and tendencies, and many of the diseases of the larynx, ear and eye. This condition of the system also renders it extremely subject (when exposed to the exciting cause) to typhoid, intermittent and remittent fevers. The vital powers are so depressed that the organism on light exposure to cold, is liable to be frostbitten and is strongly inclined to attacks of pneumonia and bronchitis, with diseases of the eye and ear.

In short, the long list of army diseases may be traced, in great measure, to an extreme susceptibility to them, which susceptibility is produced by a want of the proper admixture of nutrient ingredients in the food of the soldier in campaigns. All authorities agree that scorbutic states arise from this cause, and no one having any experience in army diseases can fail to detect symptoms of scorbutus in almost every one of them. If they are not plainly visible in the apparently well man, they make themselves manifest in him as soon as he is placed under treatment for any disease, in the surprising benefit his system derives from the vegetable acid salts of potassa and iron, and from the free use of those articles of food of which his system has been deprived. Without this treatment almost all army diseases become obstinate to deal with, much more so than similar ones in private practice.

In old cases of chronic diarrhœa, it frequently happens that the diarrhœa somewhat abates, the appetite becomes remarkably good and the patient fattens rapidly. His abdomen becomes hard and distended, it being either dropsical, tympanitic, or distended by enlarged viscera; the whole surface becomes bloated and presents the appearance of having been affected by an excessive use of alcoholic beverages. The eyes become prominent, red and watery; the thyroid glands become enlarged; the heart gives marked evidence of fibrinous depositions [1] internally,

---

[1] It has been noticed that in certain cases of heart disease the thyroid glands become enlarged, and the eyes prominent, watery and red. Whether there is any

the breathing is oppressed, and there is more or less paralytic tendency.

The same symptoms and pathological lesions, in the same order, result as have been heretofore described, and these diseases yield readily to the diet and treatment prescribed for cases of chronic diarrhœa.

Microscopic Examination of the Blood.

The purpose of the following chapter is to indicate what should be looked for in blood examinations. Also the proportion and condition of the cell elements of the blood and the knowledge which is to be gained by careful observation of the manner in which they arrange and comport themselves between the slides of the microscope. Abnormal bodies and forms in the blood, that act as specific causes of grave pathological derangements and lesions. Condition, appearance and arrangement of the fibrin filaments of the blood in health and disease. Valuable means of diagnosticating certain pathological states of the system. The fibrin in health : the fibrin in rheumatism : the fibrin in pulmonary tuberculosis : the fibrin in Anæmia. The appearance and condition of the fibrin and other blood elements, where there is tendency to the formation of Thrombi and Emboli. Finally the appearance and morphological elements of the blood, in health and in disease.

Over twenty-seven years ago, I commenced the microscopic examination of blood, with the view of arriving at positive pathological conditions and so on, in this fluid in disease. These examinations have been conducted with great care and patience, being often repeated at short intervals in the same case, in order to watch the successive changes brought about by treatment, and to confirm previous observations.

analogy between the condition of the symptom in this form of heart disease, and that productive of heart disease, chronic diarrhœa, paralytic tendencies, etc. in the army, I am unable to say. I merely mention the circumstance here to draw attention in this direction.

In this work, I have already made over eighty thousand individual examinations. In all the more important of these I have made exact drawings of the abnormal appearances and bodies present, and noted minutely the pathological conditions and the attendant symptoms and lesions.

This paper is a brief summary of a portion of this labor. It is with much hesitation that it is presented in this incomplete condition. It was my intention to work on, and to spend much more time in labors at once so interesting and so helpful to me in the treatment of disease, before making any public statement on this subject. But a few learned gentlemen, who have taken great interest in these inquiries, have earnestly requested that they be published, so that others may be induced to commence and extend investigations in the same direction.

To obtain the blood, a clean puncture or cut is made in any part of the body desired, the surface being previously cleaned with care. The wound should be large enough to allow the free and immediate escape of a drop on slight pressure. The blood is at once transferred to the slide, then quickly covered with thin glass and placed under the microscope. By a little experience, it may be placed under observation in one second from the time it leaves the blood stream.

What to look for in Blood Examinations.

Blood examinations, to be of value in diagnosis, must be made with great care. Of the microscopes in present use, not one in fifty is suited for this kind of study. They are lacking in definition and often are not sufficiently achromatic.

A drop of blood may frequently be explored for an hour or more with profit. If the case be obscure, and the first drop examined fails to throw light, explore another thoroughly. If you still fail, continue the search till you are perfectly satisfied that the cause of disease is to be sought for elsewhere. Often much may be learned by allowing the blood to stand for from a few hours to two or three days between the slides, watching from time to time the successive changes taking place during the process of drying. These changes, when compared with those taking place under similar conditions, in healthy blood, often throw valuable light upon certain peculiarities of the case.

The following is a list in detail of some of the conditions, states and pathological products to be sought for in blood.

1. Color of blood to the unaided eye and under the microscope.
2. Consistence of the blood.
3. Rapidity of clotting.
4. Serum in normal proportion.
5. Colored corpuscles in normal proportion.
6. Colorless corpuscles in normal proportion.
7. Fibrin in normal proportion.
8. Serum in too small quantity.
9. Colored corpuscles in too small quantity.
10. Colorless corpuscles in too small quantity.
11. Fibrin in too small quantity.
12. Serum in too large proportion.
13. Colored corpuscles in too large proportion.
14. Colorless corpuscles in too large proportion.
15. Fibrin in too large proportion.
16. Colored corpuscles of normal consistence.
17. Colored corpuscles too soft, plastic and sticky, adhering together and being drawn out into thread-like prolongations as they separate.
18. Colorless corpuscles normal in quantity, but so sticky and plastic that they adhere together in masses, endangering the formation of thrombi and emboli.
19. Fibrin meshes normal in size and in arrangement, allowing the free circulation of blood cells through them.
20. Fibrin meshes too small to admit of the free circulation of blood cells through them, on account of which the blood

cells arrange themselves in ropy rows, or ridges and masses, being held in the meshes of the partially clotted or contracted fibrin. In such cases the individual fibrin filaments have an increased diameter and opacity.

21. Colored corpuscles arrange themselves in nummular piles.

22. Colored corpuscles have little or no tendency to arrange themselves in nummular piles.

23. Colorless corpuscles many of them ragged, partially broken down, and more or less curled, twisted and wrinkled.

24. No tendency of the blood discs to arrange themselves in nummular piles, but remaining evenly and loosely scattered over the field.

25. The blood discs may exhibit a slight tendency to group themselves, having empty spaces between them.

26. The blood discs may arrange themselves in irregular, compact masses, occupying but a small portion of the field.

27. The blood discs may arrange themselves in ridges, exhibiting a sticky stringiness and ropiness.

28. The blood discs may hold firmly the coloring matter and be soft and plastic.

29. The blood discs may be high colored, smooth and even in outline, hard and rigid, and hold firmly and smoothly the coloring matter.

30. The blood discs may allow the coloring matter to escape readily, obscuring the individual outlines of the discs.

31. The discs may be mammillated.

32. The colorless corpuscles may be in excess or in too small quantity, and be normal in consistence.

33. The colorless corpuscles may be in excess, to a greater or lesser extent, and be sticky, plastic and adhesive, having a tendency to stick together in groups and masses. Under such circumstances, there is great danger ahead from the liability to the formation of thrombi and emboli.

34. The colorless corpuscles may be in excess, and ragged and broken.

35. The colorless corpuscles may be in excess, and smooth and even in outline.

36. Minute grains and ragged masses of black, blue, brown, or yellow pigmentary matter may occur, disseminated throughout the blood.

37. Globules and masses of fat may be present.

38. Amyloid matter may be present.

39. Masses of broken-down and disintegrating parent cells may be present.

40. Emboli of fibrin may be present in greater or lesser quantity. These emboli may or may not be filled with granular and crystalline matters.

41. Emboli of mycoderma spores may be present.

42. Filaments and spores of algæ, forming emboli, may be present.

43. Filaments and spores of algæ may be diffused or disseminated through the blood without being aggregated in masses.

44. Spores of fungi may be present.

45. Spores and filaments of fungi may be present.

46. Granules and crystals of oxalate of lime may be present.

47. Granules and crystals of cystine may be present.

48. Granules and crystals of phosphates may be present.

49. Granules and crystals of stellurine may be present.

50. Granules and crystals of stelline may be present.

51. Granules and crystals of matters of a miscellaneous character may be present.

52. Conchoidine may be present.

53. Pigmentine may be present.

54. Leucine may be present.

55. Creatine may be present.

56. The lithates or lithic acid may be present.

57. Inosite may be present.

58. Both the serum and blood discs may contain brain fat or cholesterine.

59. The blood discs only may contain brain fat.

60. The Zymotosis regularis is present in the spore state.

61. The spores and filaments of Zymotosis regularis may both be present.

62. The spores of the Entophyticus hæmactus may be present.

63. The spores and filaments of the Entophyticus hæmactus may both be present.

64. The Penicilium quadrifidum may be present, both in the spore and filamentous states of development.

65. The spores of the Mucor malignans may be present.

66. The colorless corpuscles may contain thin, bladder-like, empty cells, of various sizes, that distend them.

67. The colorless corpuscles may contain either the spores of algæ, or fungi, or both, which tend to destroy their normal contents and to distend the outside walls of the cells, so that they may be much larger than the healthy cell, and appear like sporangia.

68. The serum and colorless corpuscles may contain the spores of the crypta Syphilitica, — and in old and severe cases of tertiary syphilis, the filaments of the vegetation may be more or less present in the serum.

There are many other things to be sought for in pathological blood, which will be spoken of hereafter. I have given the foregoing list, in order to convey to the minds of those who have not conducted examinations in this direction, some idea of what to look for. The general impression is that there is nothing to be found in the blood stream but the blood elements, and it has been considered that these elements are scarcely ever, to any great extent, pathological: also that if they are so, the microscope fails to throw much light upon the subject. This is a mistake. Experience, a good microscope and a little more time and patience devoted to blood examinations, will satisfy any physician that there is more to be learned in this direction than he has ever dreamed of. The work, however, must be diligently, thoroughly and honestly performed, and with the utmost care. The more extended the knowledge of microscopic forms, of every conceivable variety, the more readily abnormal bodies are given their proper place and importance, and the more valuable in diagnosis, are such labors to the observer.

Some pathological states and products are best studied immediately after the blood is drawn, while others can be better made out after the blood has stood a longer or shorter time between the slides and has become stationary, uncovering crystalline and granular products that were at first too much enveloped in blood cells to be discoverable. Often after having worked over a drop of blood for half a day, I have discovered new forms upon reëxamination.

In the nicer microscopic explorations, we are very apt to see only those objects and conditions we are in search of, overlooking many forms and features of such marked interest that we are astonished, on their being pointed out to us, that we should have overlooked them in the extreme care we had used. The truth of this remark will come home with peculiar force to the most diligent workers in microscopic researches in new fields. The superficial observer cannot appreciate it, as he never studies out the nicer details of the individual features and forms under observation. His mind receives simply a vague impression of the general appearance, instead of grasping in detail well-defined pictures, which alone give positive and exact knowledge.

The symptoms and pathological consequences of the presence of stelline, stellurine, pigmentine and conchoidine, are briefly set forth in my paper describing these substances, published in the New York Record for February 1st, 1868. The symptoms and pathological states excited by the presence in the blood and tissues of cystine, oxalate of lime, phosphates and lithic acid, are described in my paper on Rheumatism, published in the American Journal of Medical Sciences for July and October, 1867.

The symptoms and abnormal states excited by the presence of spores and filaments of algæ and fungi, have been briefly spoken of in several of my papers, and will be more fully set forth in a paper now nearly ready. The presence of cholesterine in the blood discs of healthy blood, and in it and the serum in certain forms of disease, is the subject of another paper now ready, and which will soon appear. Other pathological states produced by abnormal conditions of the blood cells will also be comprised in a separate paper.

I will now present briefly some observations connected with

The Condition, Appearance and Arrangement of the Fibrin Filaments in the freshly drawn Blood in Health and Disease. A valuable means of diagnosticating certain pathological states of the system.

There is no possible doubt but that the fibrin filaments exist already formed in the blood stream. By a little practice, the eye can begin to explore a drop of blood under the microscope, in one second after it has left the blood stream. An experienced observer will immediately detect colorless corpuscles, masses of granules and sporoid bodies, and sometimes crystals that are fixed, or made almost stationary by some invisible means. If the eye watches these closely, while the balance of the blood is moving this way and that, and running in little currents in various directions, in a few moments, faintly delineated filaments will be noticed, forming a meshwork which holds fast these fixed cells, granules and spores. These are the fibrin filaments, which make up an almost invisible network in the freshly drawn blood. This network of organized fibrin gradually loses the almost perfect transparency it has in the blood stream, and becomes by degrees more and more opaque and visible in outline, till in the course of five or ten minutes after it is drawn, the network of threads reaches its maximum opacity, the filaments being, to the educated eye, well defined.

The fibrin filaments are developed from the fibrin cells organized in the arterial extremities of the spleen and lacteal and lymphatic glands. These cells are mostly developed into filaments before they leave the glandular capillaries. The nucleus, or " yolk " of the fibrin cells, forms the blood disc, while the portion of the cell outside of the nucleus is " spun " into a fine fibrin thread. This whole process is fully described in my paper on the " Histology and Functions of the Spleen and Lacteal and Lymphatic Glands," published in the American Journal of Medical Sciences for April, 1866.

Upon the appearance and state of the filaments and size of the meshes of this fibrin network, much depends. What might appear to be slight derangements in the parent cells that organize the fibrin cells, may result in grave pathological states. The trouble doubtless starts primarily with defective or deranged alimentation, or with some disturbance of the digestive apparatus of the alimentary canal, by which improper, defective, irritating or poisonous food is transmitted to the parent fibrin cells of the spleen and lymphatic glands. This imperfect food, little by little deranges the digesting, assimilating and organizing functions of these organisms, so that the fibrin cells manufactured by them are in one or more ways pathological. These diseased cells produce fibrin filaments that are more or less abnormal.

Now the causes that produce disturbance in the blood, may be so far removed from the pathological results at the time we detect them in the blood, that they are entirely lost in the consideration of the subject. Perhaps we only recognize the pathological products and conditions we find present in this fluid at the time of our examination, and give to these the place of *causes* of the systemic disturbance. This may be to a great extent true of them, but the physician should be able to look beyond these specific excitants, to the primary or generic causes, which have perhaps been operating for years in deranging the functions of the mother cells. This knowledge he should have, that he may be enabled to impart such instructions to his patient, after specific or immediate causes are removed, as will assist the latter to escape the danger of again falling into the same pathological state, by living in a proper manner.

Here is a field for much careful research and patient labor. It is in this direction that positive medicine may be *greatly extended* by close study and honest, persevering investigation.

Appearance and Arrangement of Fibrin Filaments in Health.

Where the system is in all respects healthy, where every part of the complicated machine performs its functions normally, the colored and colorless corpuscles are distributed evenly throughout the serum, and the fibrin meshwork does not interfere with the free movement of the blood elements. As the natural process of clotting goes on, after the blood is removed from the system, the fibrin filaments contract, decreasing the size of the meshes of the network, so that the blood elements are, to a considerable extent, caught and held fast.

If, however, the freshly drawn blood be stirred constantly with a rod till the clotting process is over, the fibrin will be found adhering to the rod in white ropes and shreds, being almost perfectly free from the colored and colorless corpuscles. The reason of this is that the blood cells, through the motion kept up in the fibrin, are washed out from the network before the filaments have contracted sufficiently to hold the blood cells fast in the fibrin meshes.

The filaments of fibrin in the healthy blood are much smaller and less strongly marked than in rheumatic and tubercular states : also the meshes of the network are larger, allowing the blood cells to pass freely through them in all directions. Fig. 1, Plate III, represents the fibrin network of healthy blood as it presents itself between the slides of the microscope, a few minutes after the blood leaves the blood stream. It will be seen that this network is free from spores, granules, colorless corpuscles and crystals. There are no abnormal products adhering to the filaments or fastened in the meshes. All the elements of the blood are normal.

Appearance and Arrangement of Fibrin Filaments in Rheumatism.

In rheumatic conditions, the filaments of the fibrin network of the blood are in a tonic state of contraction. This increases the size of the filaments, making them more plainly visible, and decreases the size of the meshes, so that the blood is in the premonitory stage of clotting, the meshes being so small that they interfere with the free passage of the blood elements — they holding in their meshes the colored and colorless corpuscles. This makes the blood have a ropy, half clotted appearance between the slides.

In a few minutes after rheumatic blood is placed between the slides, the colorless and colored corpuscles arrange themselves in ropy rows and masses, leaving large, irregular, clear spaces, in which may be distinctly traced the meshwork of fibrin filaments.

Frequently for months before the patient has any idea that he is rheumatic, or in danger of being taken suddenly down with rheumatism at any moment, this condition may be positively diagnosticated by the appearance and condition of the blood. By this mode of working, the causes of this dreaded disease may be discovered and removed before the patient is aware of his danger, thereby perhaps saving severe suffering and grave pathological disturbance.

In rheumatism, there appears to be a tendency to a tonic contraction in all the connective tissue and fibrin elements of the body. The whole muscular system is more or less stiffened and rigid. The suppleness and elasticity pertaining to the perfect physiological state are gone, and a heavy, non-elastic, more or less lame feeling pervades the organism. This tonic muscular rigidity no doubt extends to the muscular fibres of organic life, and into the walls of all hollow vessels, as those of the blood apparatus and alimentary canal. This condition, together with the tendency of the connective tissue to contract under the influence of cold, renders a rheumatic patient extremely sensitive to cold and exposure. His system usually indicates meteorological changes as swiftly as a barometer. There is a tonic state of contraction, as before said, in the fibrin filaments of the blood and in the connective tissue throughout the body: this connective tissue makes up all the tendons, fasciæ, sheaths, tubes, strings, cords, ropes and bands which connect, tie, hold, support and keep the various organs and tissues of the body in place.

This contraction and shortening of the fibrin and connective tissue filaments, arises from fermenting foods of various kinds in the digestive apparatus. This fermentation imparts to the entire organism a sour state which produces a partial clotting of the blood, and the above described tonic contraction and rigidity, which in turn narrows the calibre of all the blood-vessels and produces a general stiffening or want of elasticity in all parts of the body. Especially is this manifest after the system has been quietly resting in one position for some time. In this state, whenever the patient is exposed to cold that chills, all the connective tissues around the joints (at these places the glue tissue prevails) so contract that the calibre of the blood-vessels is so lessened that the ropy, sticky blood cannot pass or flow freely through them; in consequence the blood hangs, is partially dammed up, and congestions and inflammations arise which constitute the so-called rheumatism. These congestions are apt to take place first in the joints of those extremities which are furthest removed from the heart.

Fig. 2, Plate III, represents the appearance and condition of the fibrin network in the blood of rheumatism as exhibited in the vacant places between the slides. It will be seen that the fibrin filaments are more contracted and larger, and the meshes of the network smaller than in healthy blood. This difference is in reality more strongly marked than the drawings represent it to be.

Spores, granules, colorless corpuscles and crystals are seen fastened or caught in the network. These bodies and conditions are pathological. They are never found present in healthy blood.

Appearance and Arrangement of Fibrin Filaments in Pulmonary Tuberculosis.

In tubercular disease the blood has somewhat the appearance presented in rheumatic affections, save that there is less tendency for the colored and colorless corpuscles to become aggregated in ropy rows and masses; still the resemblance is in many cases quite strong. In tubercular phthisis there are almost always more or less flying rheumatic neuralgia pains. The fibrin filaments are sometimes almost as large and well defined and the meshes as small as in rheumatism. These pathological conditions are present for the reason that this disease is almost always accompanied with more or less of the specific causes of rheumatism. At Fig. 3, Plate III, is represented the network of fibrin filaments in pulmonary tuberculosis. The fibrin filaments are contracted and distinct, and the meshes much smaller than in health. In the meshes and sticking to the filaments are seen spores, granules, colorless corpuscles and so forth. These bodies are fastened in the fibrin network, and the conditions present, which fix and hold them, are pathological.

Appearance and Arrangements of the Fibrin Filaments in the Blood of Anæmia.

In pure cases of anæmia, that is, in states of the system where the organized histological elements of the blood are in the proper proportion, but where they exist in a quantity by far too small, — the great mass of the blood being serum, — the filaments of fibrin are small and faintly delineated, and the meshes of the network formed by them are large, allowing the thinly scattered blood elements to float freely in all directions in the serum, between the slides, without any distinct evidence of clotting. In such cases the red and white corpuscles are evenly distributed throughout the serum, there being but slight contractive tendency in the fibrin filaments; hence the meshes remain so large that they do not entangle the blood elements.

When, however, the rheumatic or tubercular diathesis accompany anæmia, then the fibrin filaments assume all the characteristics peculiar to these pathological conditions.

At Fig. 4, Plate III, is represented the network of fibrin in the blood of a pure case of anæmia.

Appearance and Condition of the Fibrin and other Blood Elements where there is a Tendency to the Formation of Thrombi and Emboli.

Whenever there exist in the blood abnormal bodies which are insoluble in the serum, more or less irritation of the living tissue of the blood apparatus — especially in the heart and its vicinity — is the result. Sooner or later the organic muscular fibres lose a part of their tonicity, and there are frequently tired feelings, wandering pains and aches, which are more prone to hang about the cardiac region than elsewhere. The insoluble matters floating in the blood have a tendency to fix themselves — in or near the heart — to the epithelial lining, whose secretions then assume a more or less plastic and sticky condition from the irritation excited. These fixed fibres become centres for the gradual accretions of fibrin, which applies itself slowly, layer upon layer, and finally, little by little, we have formed thrombi. From time to time these break loose from their points of attachment and float as emboli in the blood stream.

There is also another condition of the blood elements where there is great danger of thrombosis and embolism, and which may be readily diagnosticated by means of the microscope, in time to avert those serious results which may await the patient. This is *stickiness* and *plasticity* of the fibrin filaments and colorless corpuscles. The stickiness often extends even to the blood discs. Whenever this state is present the colorless corpuscles, instead of being scattered about singly, are found sticking together in groups of two, three, four or more.

The fibrin filaments are also sticky and plastic, and impede the free flow of the blood cells through their network. The result is a marked tendency to the formation of thrombi and emboli.

Emboli under such conditions are frequently produced simply by the sticking together of the colorless corpuscles, forming masses of greater or lesser size. They are also formed by the breaking loose of thrombi. This sticky state of the blood is usually scorbutic, and arises mainly from deranged or defective alimentation.

In conclusion I would say that this chapter is but an imperfect brief of extended labors in this direction.

XLVI.

PLAN OF TREATING DISEASE.

THE first and most important knowledge of which a physician should possess himself is a thorough and detailed understanding of all the appearances, symptoms and conditions of the body which constitute a perfect state of health. Without this he is unable to determine, locate and measure the derangements which constitute disease. He should know the microscopic appearance, density and color of healthy urine, and the quantity that should be passed daily; also its chemical composition. He should know the color of healthy blood when first drawn, its consistence, activity and microscopic appearance, or the picture it presents when highly magnified. Any departure in its appearance or condition from the healthy state, indicates some form of disease. The slighter the variation, the more readily the physician should detect and interpret it; the nearer he comes to arresting the disease in its incipient stages, the more speedy will be the cure. He should guard himself against the prevalent error of an irresponsible age, blind to all but surface indications. He should be quick to recognize those deep laid, preparatory plans of disease, or the first meditated departure of the system from normal conditions, as indicated by slight but unmistakable changes in blood, urine, stools and secretions. He should perfectly understand what constitutes healthy digestion, healthy stools and healthy states of all the various membranes and glands, that he may instantly discover the first deviation from health. The hair follicles, sweat and fat glands, and epidermic surfaces in their best states and moods should be closely studied and wholly known. The same may be said of all other parts of the body : he must master every detail of the wonderful human machine which he proposes to repair and restore. He should not content himself with the recognition of established disease in its earlier forms, but should detect it, so to say, in embryo.

In handling disease, or any departure from the healthy state, the first thing to determine is the kind, character, extent and peculiarity of the derangements ; the histological elements ; the organs and the tissues involved, and finally the cause or causes that are operating to produce (and are at the very bottom of) all the trouble. These points accurately determined, the way is opened for removing such cause or causes and restoring healthy conditions.

We will suppose that a patient presents himself for treatment : you find him having chilly feelings during the forenoon, fever during the afternoon, and profuse cold sweats at and during the night. He has a severe cough ; the pulse is weak and frequent ; urine scanty (about one quart daily), very high colored, and standing at a density of 1.030 : he is weak, his heart palpitates on exertion and he is much shrunken and emaciated, especially about the chest. If the sputa be examined with the microscope it is found more or less filled with shreds of broken-down connective tissue. The stomach and bowels are filled with fermenting foods ; the patient is flatulent and may have morning diarrhœa, though often they are constipated. This is a case of consumption in the last or breaking-down stage, as more fully described in previous chapters. The patient is dying faster than he is living. Digestion and assimilation are very poor and consequently blood and tissue are not made fast enough to keep pace with decay and disintegration. The processes of death are on the track with the agencies and efforts of life. It is a race, and Death is neck and chest ahead ! If nothing can be done to retard him and accelerate the processes of life and repair, the end soon comes, and the race is honestly won by Death.

Something can be done. This something lies first in the

direction of improving digestion, assimilation, blood-making and repair of tissue. On close examination the digestive organs are found full of the products of fermenting vegetable foods, breads, fruits and sweets. Both alcoholic and acid fermentations are present in full force. There is but little digestion and assimilation of food.

The first step is to wash out the sour stomach and bowels, and to change the food. The food selected should be such as is least liable to ferment with alcohol and acid yeasts. This is the muscle pulp of beef, prepared as heretofore described, when it affords the maximum of nourishment with the minimum of effort to the digestive organs. *Nothing else* but this food, except an occasional change to broiled mutton.

The washing should be done one hour and a half before each meal and half an hour before retiring, as previously directed in this work. Usually a pint of hot water at each drinking is about the quantity required to wash out the slimy stomach, and to get it clean and free enough from bile and yeasty matter to digest lean meats. The water must be taken slowly at first, as it may nauseate if taken too rapidly. Should it nauseate, sprinkle in a little salt, or put in a small quantity of clear tea or coffee, or half a teaspoonful of aromatic spirits of ammonia.

In a day or two the urine will begin to flow more freely. This indicates the cleansing of the stomach. The stools become black and tarry, the bile being washed down through the bowels instead of passing off through the kidneys. If this washing and eating are persisted in, the urine keeps getting lighter in color and greater in quantity from day to day, till in the course of a couple of weeks or so it has become as clear as an infant's, stands at a density of from 1.010 to 1.015, and flows at the rate of from sixty-four to eighty ounces daily. The stomach is now clean, the appetite for meat good; digestion and assimilation are so far improved that blood is made faster than it is used up, and repair of tissue is going on. Chills, fever and sweats have either ceased or are rapidly growing lighter and the cough is greatly better. The cure has begun. The life processes have now the advantage over those of death, and if care be taken to avoid all departures and accidents, Life, on "the home stretch," wins, and the patient is well. It takes almost three years — sometimes more — to effect a perfect cure, when the patients are in this last stage of the disease. Natural processes are slow but sure, and this cure follows closely the course indicated by Nature. To cleanse all the organs and render the system a fit receptacle for a healthy blood stream; to purify that blood stream and keep it steadily flowing, in its normal condition, through the diseased organism which it repairs, — this follows the hint given us by Nature when the wound of the healthy savage heals far more rapidly than that of the man of civilization, or when the least scratch may fester on the scrofulous child, which on its playmate has no effect beyond a moment's pain. "Blood is the great arcanum of Life." When you have cleansed out the system and purified the blood, keep them so and hope all things. There should be no hurry. Calm, passive and faithful following out of all instructions to the letter will insure the life and health of the patient, if with soul and body equally enlisted in the cause he treads this "straight and narrow way."

If the patient, from accident or any other cause, loses the appetite for meat, the urine will be found higher colored, and the stomach dirty and containing bile. This condition may have been caused by poor meat (badly broiled or immature beef, etc.), and be entirely accidental and unavoidable; or it may be caused by tasting food outside of the lines laid down; by over-exertion, excitement, or by want of proper rest before and after eating. Whatever the cause, draw the lines tightly, wash more vigorously, lessen the amount eaten, select the meat with care, and hold strictly to the lean beef, prepared in the nicest manner and fairly well done. Rare meat is not good for the consumptive; fairly well done meat digests more readily and does more good.

In a few days the appetite for the meat returns, when digestion and assimilation improve. The urine becomes clear, the stomach is clean and all goes on well again.

In the cases of patients who do not like the meat, it is well to call their attention from the mere taste on the palate, to their comfortable condition after eating, and the glow which spreads through the system. If they do not then like it, this is either because they do not want to do so, or because they have tasted or even smelled other food at the table where persons not under treatment were eating. The imagination is a powerful factor in this matter, and sometimes a relish for the meat does not come until the palate (to put it that way) has forgotten the taste of accustomed foods. Hence the importance of not even tasting or considering the forbidden, apart from the other fact that one mouthful may suffice to start up fermentation, just as a handful of "mother" from an old vinegar barrel serves as a basis for acetic fermentation in the new and sweet one.

During the early part of the treatment, while the patient is weak and sweating, it is well to bathe night and morning with hot water in which a tablespoonful of strong aqua ammonia is added to the quart, after which rub in all over the following mixture : —

R/	Alcohol	.	.	.	.	.	.	.	.	.	℥xv
	Quinina Sulph. .		.	.	.	.	.	.	.	ℨiss	
	Acid Sulphuric		.	.	.	.	.	.	ℨi		
	Pure Glycerine		.	.	.	.	.	℥i.	*M.*		

Before each meal a teaspoonful of a good tonic, something like the following, should be given : —

R/	Pure Glycerine	.	.	.	.	.	.	℥i
	Fluid Extract Anise .		.	.	.	.	℥ss
	" " Caraway .		.	.	.	.	℥ss
	" " Hydrastis .		.	.	.	.	℥i
	" " Mullein .		.	.	.	.	℥ii
	" " Elecampagne		.	.	.	.	℥iss

Fluid Extract Cinchona Comp. . . . . . ℥iss
    "   "   Guarana. . . . . . . ℥iss
    "   "   Wild Cherry . . . . . ℥i
    "   "   Hop . . . . ℥i
    "   "   Prickly Ash . . . . . ℥ss
Oil Menth. Pip. . . . . gtt xii
Sodium Bromide . . . . ℥ss. *M.*

S. Take a teaspoonful in water before each meal.

And after meals the following : —

℞   Pure Calf Pepsin . . . . ℥ii
    Pure Pancreatine . . . . ℥i
    Subnitrate Bismuth . . . . . . ℥i

  Mix and rub together well.

S. Take fifteen grains after each meal in a little water.

Keep the bowels open once daily. If constipated, take enough Epsom salts in the warm water before breakfast to give one movement. If too loose, take a teaspoonful of the following mixture in a little water two hours after each meal and on retiring : —

℞   Fluid Extract Witch Hazel . . . . . ℥vi
    "   "   Blackberry Root . . . . . ℥ii
    "   "   Cinnamon . . . . . ʒii
    "   "   Anise . . . . ʒii
    "   "   Caraway . . . . . ʒii
    "   "   Aromatic . . . . . ʒii
    Pure Glycerine . . . . ℥i
    Oil Menth. Pip. . . . . gtt x. *M.*

If the passages are still too frequent, and the bowels flatulent and disturbed with colic pains, lessen gradually the amount eaten at each meal until the flatulence and colic pains cease; and very likely by this time the diarrhœa will have ceased also. As soon as all is going on well, and one easy movement of the bowels takes place daily, without twinges of colic, the amount eaten may be little by little increased, always leaving off just before the appetite is quite satisfied.

Never mind the shrinkage in weight. It is natural and absolutely necessary, for the reason that those foods which upholster, or make fat, are the very ones which produce the disease. The weight decrease is not at all dangerous nor alarming, when from the blood examinations it is readily seen that the blood is constantly improving in quality and increasing in quantity. The patient will begin to make new and firm, healthy tissue at a later stage of his cure, when normal blood-making processes are fully restored. The tissue with which he has parted — devitalized and enervated — is no loss and must give place to that of the new order of things.

In the first days of treatment the patient often feels very feeble, owing to the absence of the artificial stimulus of fermenting foods; this also is natural and need evoke no anxieties. A cleansing process is not per se a strengthening one, but is needful in order to prepare a basis for the acquirement of real strength.

The urine should be examined daily, and kept as nearly as possible at a density of 1.010 to 1.015. The color should also be noted with care. It should be that of the urine of a healthy infant, free from bile and from the brown-yellow hue which bile confers.

Should the skin at any time become too dry and feverish, it must be daily oiled with a mixture of glycerine and water, or with vaseline or oil of sweet almonds. This should be rubbed in well after bathing.

The passages from the bowels will be black, tarry and rather small in quantity for several months. This must be expected. These dark and sticky stools are caused by the washing down of the black bile which has previously been saturating the system and being partially carried off through the urinary organs and sweat glands. The black condition of the biliary secretions is the outcome of long-continued fermentation of foods, in the stomach and bowels, keeping up constant reversed peristaltic action in the digestive organs, gall bladder and gall ducts, and culminating in a semi-paralyzed state of all the nerves which go to the portal system. There is in consequence an increased, gelatinous, adhesive condition of the secretions of the biliary apparatus and other secreting membranes and follicles which have become paralyzed in part, just as the bronchial secretions become sticky and tough in Asthma. The smallness of the passages is due to the meat foods being nearly all utilized in nourishing the body. The cleansing of stomach and intestines progresses in this slow, steady manner under favorable circumstances. In some cases, however, patients are from time to time subject to " scourings," or the passage of a number of cleansing stools daily. Such stools are often composed in large part of greenish or yellow mucus, occasionally streaked with blood. Sometimes beef-red pieces of thickened mucus are washed away from the intestinal surfaces. These must not be mistaken for the elongated folds of thickened intestine which slough off when those organs begin to take on healthy action after being cleansed by the use of hot water.[1]

The " scourings " occur from time to time at gradually lengthening intervals, growing less in quantity and severity as the intervening period grows longer, until at last the healthy stools will only attest their occurrence by a slight coating of white, coagulated mucus, looking like a fold of tissue-paper around the consolidated feces. The mucus is coagulated by the acid fermentations in the large bowels, producing acid so concentrated that it coagulates the mucus coating the inside of the

---

[1] These thickened folds, if extensive, on account of their low state of vitality (being very poorly supplied with nerves and blood-vessels) often die, decay and slough away. In this case they produce very foetid stools and prostrate the system by the poisonous effects of the decaying and disintegrating tissue. These dead folds may hang, attached to the inside of the colon, for weeks before they break loose and come away. They are in size from half an inch to a foot long, and from an eighth of an inch to an inch or more in diameter. Unless great care be taken to keep up the patient's strength and to disinfect the bowels, death may occur from sheer exhaustion.

bowel. This peels off in thin sheets, and comes away rolled up in long strings or thin, folded laminæ. The patient feels weaker during and after these scourings, which are usually attended with pain, and is sometimes very tender about the abdomen and intestines, owing to the absorption of the gases formed, which partially paralyzes the parts, resulting in neuralgic aches: also to the premature removal of thickenings, leaving the underlying surfaces somewhat irritated, as any wound is apt to be upon the abrupt removal of a scab. The cleansing process is in itself right and natural; these matters must all be washed out of the system. Yet these "scourings" are premature in the sense that they would not come to such a sudden "climax" if the patient had not been mentally wrought up and disturbed. It is quite possible to cleanse gradually, washing down these collects by slow action, and so avoid these sharp turns, provided the patient can be kept in that passive contentment which reserves the vital energies for organic uses and necessities. It is the want of this nerve-force which conduces to violent, cumulative effort in the organs struggling to throw off disease. If they receive their daily supply, they make their daily advance without friction. To this end, proscribe all undue physical and mental effort. The body from waist to thighs should be protected by knit lamb's-wool jerseys, both day and night. These should be soft and elastic, and thick enough to keep the body at a warm and even temperature, uninfluenced by the changes in weather.

If the patient's strength should be failing fast, despite of the cautious measures heretofore laid down, quinine, salicine and the pure liquors — whiskey, brandy, gin and rum — may be given in such doses as best agree with the patient. The liquors should be old, and cured well in wood for ten or more years, or biliousness may be produced by the fusel oil which they contain. In some cases the liquors will become acid in a few moments after reaching the stomach; in such instances they should be avoided. Prohibit them also whenever they heighten the color of the urine.

Bear well in mind that nothing which heightens the color of the urine or lessens the appetite for meat should be given. The moment any permitted departure on the part of the patient is found to impede his progress in any one direction, he must at once be brought back to strict dietetic principles.

The subject of further derangements in the course of the cure will be more fully considered in the following chapter.

XLVII.

THE RELATIONS OF PATIENT AND PHYSICIAN.   THEIR BEARING UPON THE CURE.

In the course of treatment, drawbacks and upsets frequently arise in the cases of patients who have not at once accepted the system with full and cheerful conviction. These retard and complicate the cure.

There is no fixed routine, no " cast-iron rule " in this respect. Were I to detail some such drawbacks, the student would think that the whole synopsis lay formulated before him; he would not bring his individual judgment, his trained and acute observation to bear upon these varying disturbances. They are as different in kind as are individuals; there are almost as many of them as there are patients. Each and all of these peculiar drawbacks arise from the condition of the patient's mind, from something he has thought or done, when they are not caused by dietetic or other infringements of rule. Perhaps he lacks faith in the system, in his physician, in himself. Then he daily convenes a debating society in his cerebrum, and exhausts his vital energy by useless mental operations. He weighs the pros and cons of his treatment and whether he did well to begin it; he magnifies and collects the idle remarks of his acquaintances as to his emaciation, or a superior method, or what not. This debating and arguing are senseless after he has once begun and is actually pursuing the course, however valid it may have been before entering upon the treatment. He should be made to understand that these nervous and unbalanced states react upon the diseased organs in many unfavorable ways, by depriving them of that sympathetic nervous force which alone completes perfectly normal action.

In this respect also it is needful to go to the root of the trouble, to seek out the Cause. That Cause is bound up in the relations of physician and patient and in the duty owed by each to each. It is first of all necessary that the patient should have full trust in the physician and the methods employed, if he is to avoid the insane friction of a mind " divided against itself." The physician in his turn must be worthy of this trust. " Faith without works is dead." Faith alone cannot restore diseased organs. On the other hand, while we may purify the blood and repair the system, this is still insufficient ; if we cannot supply the organism with increased vital force we have an engine without steam. The patient, debilitated and often hypochondriacal, depends largely upon the physician for this force at the start, since he and he only can awaken the sick man's dormant confidence and teach him how to save and accumulate vital energy, as I shall subsequently demonstrate.

The physician should understand most thoroughly his patient's condition and disease, and should take an accurate and full measure of the case. He should have a clear conception of the best mode of procedure and an abiding faith in the only and best course to be taken to effect the best results. His mental serenity and scientific security will be felt by the patient, who will rest in and upon them without himself knowing why he does so.

The physician should be as transparent as glass to his patient, and explain fully all present conditions and states, and the only ways and means which offer a chance for recovery, together with the reasons for the same. He should amply demonstrate that the success of the efforts towards health rests largely and mainly with the patient, who has the power to arrest improvement not by deeds alone, but by enfeebling, useless thought ; for this reason he should above all be honest and sincere with himself.

The patient should realize that no man can do for him what he will not do for himself. No other can so truly befriend

him. Mechanical obedience is but one half the battle ; the patient must not only will, he must believe. The whole nature of
man must be brought to the task, moral as well as physical,
for the seat of disease is not confined to the body ; the vital
energies are wasted ; the will, often the mind, are impaired.
Fidelity of the body is as nothing if not reinforced by fidelity
of the soul.

The patient should keep a strict register of all he does and
balance accounts every day, confessing fully to himself all his
sins of omission and commission. He must remember that he
himself has established these diseased states by complete absorption in mistaken habits of living during a long period of years,
and that he must in reason expect to employ some time, and an
equal interest, in retracing his steps towards health. He must
place the keystone on the arch, or all the building of the physician is comparatively vain. This keystone is a passive serenity, an intimate and abiding faith in himself, in his ability to
get well and his having chosen the right course to pursue in
this direction.

The physician, in all his relations towards his patient, should
manifest a sincere, calm, passive and whole-souled deportment,
such as always inspires confidence. If the patient gets excited,
blames, worries or finds fault, he will know at once that the sick
man has been transgressing, and is out of order, — unbalanced
physically first, and mentally and morally afterward. Now is
the time for the physician to be passive, firm and kind. His
words should be uttered firmly, gently, slowly, and always to the
point. His motions should also be slow, decided, and his whole
demeanor full of confidence in the right course. If he feels
this within himself, and has withal that boundless compassion
and desire to cure which alone carry a man through such ar-
duous labors and thorough medical training as I have herein indicated, — if he feels all this he can radiate it out to his patient
through every pore, in every gesture and tone. His life-force,
his personal magnetism are in all these, as he charges them

with peace and good-will. Man acts upon man at every point and most of all at the guidance of his inner conviction. He who does not feel this will never be a true healer : he cannot impart what he does not possess, and without the energies inspired by faith and hope the work is incomplete, as my experience has shown. Let the physician therefore assure his patient that if he would get well he must have confidence in himself and in the sure results of right doing, which cannot fail in the end. The cure depends almost wholly upon the acts, and mental and moral sincerity of the patient. This must be stamped upon his mind and heart. A course of this kind soon quiets and fortifies the patient and impresses him with a sense of his individual responsibility. Held to such an account, he has a right to expect a return in kind from his physician, as well as an exhaustive and detailed knowledge to which Therapeutics must come before it can deserve the name.

XLVIII.

STOPPING THE LEAKS IN VITAL ENERGY, SO AS TO SAVE AND ACCUMULATE VITALITY IN THE BODY.

AFTER having quite successfully traced nearly every disease to its cause, and finding myself able to build up the body and get it apparently in a good physical condition, there was one very important element wanting to effect a perfect cure. This was my inability to get vitality into the system as fast as it was put in physiological repair. Many times my patients would reach an apparently healthy condition, but would have little power to exert themselves : often they would feel quite well and yet have little or no muscular endurance.

For a long time my mind dwelt upon this point with a persistent determination to fathom the mystery. I went to my library one evening after dinner, — first giving orders that I should not be disturbed on any account whatsoever, — locked the door, partially lowered the light, and seated myself in an easy-chair, with my eyes fixed vacantly upon the gray wall of the ceiling, and dropped back mentally into myself, contemplating passively and attentively the sensations and workings in every part of the body.

I had not been in this contemplative mood more than fifteen minutes, before I found myself thrilled through and through with a glow of healthy, happy action in every part that was in purest sense most delightful. I remained in this state for about two hours, which were the happiest my life had ever known up to that time. I felt the coming and going of that indefinable yet potent soul-force which shapes and forms the human frame, which stands behind our will like the power behind the throne:

I had observed it at its work, and felt its secret and energic springs. At the end I found myself greatly strengthened and in a most happy glow all over, because I had for the time made myself passively receptive to the influx of this power, laying aside mere will and desire, but waiting as the Greeks said the "soul waits upon the gods." I had taken in life largely, and my whole system, physical and mental, felt greatly invigorated. It came to me then that I had solved one step in the process of holding and accumulating life : that the reason why we are often so exhausted, is that we are constantly wasting energy in meaningless mental and physical operations which have no useful outcome, bettering neither others nor ourselves. The way to accumulate and store up this life-force is to stop throwing it away.

Nearly every evening for several months I kept up this study upon myself for two or three hours at a time, in order to work out the problem with sufficient accuracy, so that I might impart to my sick patients the ways and means of accumulating life-force. I found that all mechanical efforts, whether mental or physical, exhaust and deplete us of energy faster than we can take it in, while all enjoyable and inspirational pursuits invigorate; that is, in these last energy or life-force is taken in faster than it is expended. This difference arises from the mental conditions under which we act, and which in turn react upon the physical organs and affect physical conditions favorably or the reverse. In the case of inspirational action every part of ourselves is interested and occupied without division or strain, while in automatic pursuits the operations are performed mechanically and with undue friction, or we reach feverishly and frantically for unprofitable ends which, attained, satiate and weary us ; misled as we are by the erratic workings of an overtaxed cerebrum, we pass our lives in casting life away. Perfect harmony of action in the entire man invigorates every part. He gives freely and receives more than he expends. By inspirational acts, I mean those acts to which we feel prompted from within, and which seem to be the natural outcome of our life, so that we move along easily with them, as with a strong current, to success.

Thus we should as far as possible avoid all mechanical efforts, and engage only in congenial and interesting pursuits. The idle ramblings of an exaggerated fancy, or the senseless worries of morbid anxieties weaken the mind; the automatic efforts of a listless body drain it of life-force. This is especially manifest and proven true in handling disease. If patients go into this treatment saying " damn " to it back in their minds, at every step; although they may have the will to carry out the system to the utmost letter, there will be no true recovery. The sympathetic nerves, the soul-nerves, the forces which run the body when we are asleep as well as awake, — these must be interested in the good work. Faith must anneal the whole. Then the double processes of repair and gain go on rapidly and with entire satisfaction to both physician and patient. The stomach gets clean, the urine clear, the blood pure, the appetite good; there are no dreams even of forbidden food. The patient becomes enthused, he is in the work soul and body; it is an inspirational and interesting work to him and not chain labor; he accumulates more life-force than he gives, although he feels generous and like extending to all a helping hand.

I must not be misunderstood as saying that a patient cannot be cured if his professional or other work is uncongenial to him. That is a misfortune, a drain, and many men are so placed. There is then all the more reason for teaching him how to escape from the worst effect of such labors, by learning to retreat within himself, where serenity may always be found, and to warn him from converting his treatment into just such another vexing labor. Let him learn by the weariness of that experience to make a pleasure of his cure. The moment you can make a patient understand these facts, not alone with his reason, but with the full and hearty acceptance of his soul, you have him where you can surely cure him upon this system.

In the first two chapters of this work I have indicated some simple means of getting the patient into the passive, reposeful state, and his physician or he himself may discover many others. A study of the vital centres and the manner in which the life principle is stored in them and works through them, will largely repay attention. If the man will drop back within himself and live from within outwards, not rushing out in manifold directions, but serenely selecting those external acts and inner thoughts which best express him and are most natural to his higher perceptions; if he will do his work for its own integral sake, undisturbed by worries over its results (for the majestic ordering of results lies beyond him); if he will live at the true heart of every hour as it comes to him, — then he may accumulate vital energy while freely using it, sure that he will receive in even larger ratio. " Compound interest is the rate of this exchequer." Taught by his physician to unite soul and body in his amendment with quiet but happy accord, Health will soon be for him a realization, and not a fugitive dream. And if I be asked what rightful place the soul has in a physiological work, I reply: The place it has in the Actual, the place it has in Nature. It stands within the body, evolving and using forces : it completes, organizes, governs through its henchman, the life principle, that vivifying agent without which we drop out of sight into the teeming earth. To contemplate the restoration of the man without taking into account the equilibrium of this force, is like proposing to raise the dead when once its subtle current has been breathed back into the Unseen. It may indeed work its harmonizing way without our knowledge of its aid : it may also be distraught, and the body patched up without its accord will add another ethical Frankenstein to those who stalk abroad amid our " civilization." The true healer will wisely appeal to this natural law of coöperation; he will strive to get a grasp of his patient's mind and to polarize this substanding force by the action of his own inner power.

XLIX.

EXPERIMENTS WITH "BAKED BEANS" AS AN EXCLUSIVE DIET,
UPON STRONG HEALTHY MEN.

In September, 1856, I engaged six strong, healthy men, in
the vigor of life, ranging in age from 25 to 40 years, to feed
upon a special line of diet solely, with the understanding that
I would pay them $30 per month each, if they submitted faith-
fully to the rigid discipline laid down.   At the same time I ex-
plained to them the kind of food upon which I should require
them to live, the exercise and other regulations marked out.
All thought the diet and drinks could be easily endured, in
fact, enjoyed, especially as they would have no manual labor
to perform.   They all entered upon the undertaking with the
feeling that they would have a fine time at my expense.   The
diet consisted first of baked beans and coffee.   This to continue
for one month or until otherwise ordered by me.   Exercise to
be a two-mile walk, morning and evening.   To retire at 9 p. m.
and rise at 6 a. m.   Drinks between meals, cold water.

On the 13th of September, the experiments began.   Breakfast at 7 a. m., dinner at 12 noon, and supper at 6 p. m.   I shall
designate my six boarders by the letters A, B, C, D, E, F.   All
were strong, robust, free from disease, and having one regular
movement of the bowels every day.

A	weighed	160 lbs.	Age 36 yrs.
B	"	145 "	" 30 "
C	"	155 "	" 40 "
D	"	166 "	" 34 "
E	"	172 "	" 28 "
F	"	148 "	" 25 "

The first day all felt well and enjoyed themselves greatly.

Towards evening began to bloat, but had no special feeling of discomfort. Slept well. Entered upon the second day feeling about as well as on the first, except that all were flatulent and constipated. Yet all had a scanty, hard movement of the bowels before evening. In the after part of the day they were very uncomfortable from the bloating. Took them on a brisk walk of two miles, which was something of a relief.

The following table shows the condition from the third to the eighteenth day inclusive, during which time they continued the before-mentioned diet and drinks.

DAY.	A.	B.	C.
3	Bloated badly. Constipated.	Bloated badly. Colic pains. Constipated.	Bloated badly. Colic. Constipated.
4	Badly bloated. Constipated. Movement with much wind.	Bloated badly. Colic. Slight movement with much wind.	Bloated badly. Colic. Slight movement; much wind passed.
5	Bloated badly. Constipated. Passed wind freely. Colic.	Bloated badly. Colic. Constipated. Dizzy. Bewildered.	Bloated badly. Constipated. Colic. Dizzy. Confused.
6	Bloated badly. Constipated. Ears ring. Dizzy. Colic.	Bloated badly. Colic. Constipated. Ears ring. Dizzy.	Bloated badly. Constipated. Ears ring. Dizzy. Passed much wind.
7	Bloated badly. Slight movement. Ears ring. Dizzy. Colic. Confused.	Bloated badly. Severe colic pains. Ears ring. Dizzy. Constipated.	Bloated badly. Constipated. Colic. Dizzy. Ears ring. Bewildered.
8	Bloated badly. Constipated. Ears ring. Dizzy. Passed much wind. Uneasy.	Bloated badly. Dizzy. Constipated. Passed wind freely. Confused. Ears ring.	Bloated badly. Slight movement with wind. Ears ring. Dizzy. Feels strangely.
9	Bloated badly. Constipated. Ears ring. Dizzy. Hands and feet prickle.	Bloated badly. A profuse thin passage with much wind. Dizzy. Ears ring.	Bloated badly. Constipated. Hands and feet prickle. Dizzy. Bewildered.
10	Bloated badly. Constipated. Dizzy. Hands and feet prickle. Ears ring. Strange.	Bloated badly. 2 profuse stools with wind. Feels easier. Dizzy. Ears ring.	Bloated badly. 1 profuse passage. Dizzy. Feels strange. Feet prickle.
11	1 profuse passage. Flatulent. Dizzy. Much bewildered.	3 large stools. Flatulent. Dizzy. Ears ring. Feels strangely.	2 profuse stools. Flatulent. Feels numb. Ears ring.
12	2 large stools. Feels better. Ears ring. Dizzy. Feet prickle.	5 large, thin movements. Ears ring. Dizzy. Feels strangely.	3 large stools. Feels lost. Head dizzy. Feet and hands prickle.
13	4 profuse stools. Hands numb. Head dizzy. Feels strangely.	7 large stools. Feels weak and strangely. Feet prickle.	4 profuse stools. Walks as if drunk. Feet prickle. Strange.
14	6 thin, large stools. Head vacant. Eyes staring. Feels strangely.	9 large stools. Feels drunk and weak in legs. Gait unsteady. Numb. Reels in walking.	6 large stools. Dizzy. Head numb. Ears ring. Legs and feet numb. Gait unsteady.

DAY	A.	B.	C.
15	8 thin large stools. Dizzy. Walks with difficulty. Ears ring. Feels drunk and lost.	11 large, thin stools. Feels weak and strange. Hands and feet prickle.	9 large, thin stools. Ears ring. Staggers in walking.
16	9 large, yeasty stools. Head feels empty. Tired and strange. Walks unsteady.	11 large yeasty stools. Dizzy. Head empty and strange. Hips, feet and legs numb. Feet drag.	8 large, yeasty stools. Feet and hands prickle. Bewildered. Gait unsteady. Reels in walking.
17	7 large, yeasty stools. Ears ring. Feet and hands prickle. Legs and feet numb. Gait unsteady.	12 large, thin, yeasty stools. Feels very weak and bewildered. Feet and legs numb. Walk unsteady.	10 large, yeasty stools. Ears ring. Dizzy. Weak. Reels in walking.
18	10 thin, yeasty stools. Dizzy. Bewildered. Strange. Heart palpitates on exertion. Very unsteady in gait. Feet and legs numb.	13 thin, yeasty stools. Ears ring. Dizzy. Hands and feet prickle. Heart palpitates and breathing short on any exertion. Feet and legs numb. Walks with difficulty.	12 thin, yeasty stools. Dizzy. Weak. Reels in walking. Feet drag. Feels empty and strange. Breathing begins to be oppressed. Heart pains.

DAY	D.	E.	F.
3	Bloated badly. Constipated. Ears ring. Dizzy.	Bloated badly. Slight movement. Ears ring. Dizzy.	Bloated badly. Slight movement. Colic pains. Head swims.
4	Bloated badly. Slight movement with much wind. Ears ring. Dizzy.	Bloated badly. Constipated. Colic. Ears ring. Confused.	Bloated badly. Constipated. Colic. Ears ring. Bewildered.
5	Bloated badly. Slight movement. Passed wind freely. Ears ring.	Bloated badly. Constipated. Ears ring. Bewildered. Colic.	Bloated badly. Constipated. Colic. Ears ring. Confused.
6	Bloated badly. Constipated. Colic. Ears ring. Confused.	Bloated badly. Constipated. Ears ring. Colic. Dizzy. Bewildered.	Bloated badly. Constipated. Dizzy. Colic. Confused. Uneasy and restless.
7	Bloated badly. Constipated. Dizzy. Ears ring. Passed wind.	Bloated badly. Constipated. Ears ring. Some deafness. Colic. Dizzy.	Bloated badly. Constipated. Ears ring. Dizzy. Uneasy and bewildered.
8	Bloated badly. Constipated. Dizzy. Ears ring. Feels strangely.	Bloated badly. Slight movement. Ears ring. Feels lost and strange. Feet go to sleep.	Bloated badly. Constipated. Ears ring. Dizzy. Hands and feet prickle. Bewildered.
9	Bloated badly. Thin movement with wind. Hands and feet prickle. Dizzy.	Bloated badly. Profuse, thin movement with wind. Colic. Ears ring. Dizzy.	Bloated badly. Constipated. Dizzy. Hands and feet prickle. Feels strangely and confused.
10	2 profuse movements. Flatulent. Dizzy. Hands and feet prickle.	Bloated badly. Constipated. Feels lost. Hands and feet prickle.	Bloated badly. Ears ring. Constipated. Hands and feet numb. Feels strangely.
11	4 large, thin movements. Head feels empty. Feet prickle.	2 profuse stools. Ears ring. Dizzy. Eyes staring. Feet prickle.	1 large, thin movement. Colic. Dizzy. Feet prickle. Strange.
12	5 large, thin stools. Ears ring. Confused. Feet prickle.	4 large, thin stools. Walks as if intoxicated. Feet and hands prickle.	3 large stools. Head numb and vacant. Feels lost and strange. Feet prickle.
13	6 large stools. Ears ring. Reels in walking. Confused.	5 large stools. Feels weak and exhausted. Dizzy. Ears ring.	6 large, thin stools. Forgetful and feels strangely. Feet and hands prickle. Dizzy.

DAY	D.	E.	F.
14	5 large, thin stools. Dizzy. Ears ring. Feels intoxicated.	5 large, thin stools. Feels numb and strange. Ears ring. Feet and hands prickle. Legs and feet numb.	7 large, thin stools. Ears ring. Feet and hands numb. Feels strange and vacant. Legs and feet numb.
15	10 large, thin stools. Ears ring. Feels light headed. Legs numb.	8 large, thin stools. Hands and feet prickle. Feels strangely.	10 large, thin stools. Reels in walking. Feels tired and strange.
16	11 thin, yeasty stools. Head dizzy. Ears ring. Bewildered.	9 thin, yeasty stools. Ears ring. Feels weak and vacant. Legs numb.	10 large, yeasty stools. Bewildered. Weak. Eyes vacant. Feet prickle.
17	9 thin, yeasty stools. Ears ring. Reels in walking.	8 thin, yeasty stools. Dizzy. Ears ring. Hands and feet prickle. Feet and legs numb and drag in walking.	9 thin, yeasty stools. Bewildered. Eyes vacant and glaring. Feet and hands prickle. Feet drag in walking.
18	11 thin stools. Feels numb all over. Weak and smothering feeling at times. Walks with difficulty. Feet drag.	10 thin stools. Feels weak and bewildered. Begins to feel as if he could not breathe freely. Feet drag. Cannot walk straight. Legs and hips numb.	12 thin stools. Reels in walking. Ears ring. Feet and hands numb. Nervous. Heart palpitates on exertion and breathing oppressed. Legs and hips numb. Feet drag in walking.

Symptoms of Progressive Paralysis or Locomotor Ataxy began to show themselves in all six cases on tenth day. These paralytic and peculiar symptoms increased each day after the tenth. On sixteenth day the disease was so marked, that not one of the six could walk straight without support. All wobbled and dragged their legs, not being able to lift them clear of the floor.

Diet changed to Meats.

DAY	A.	B.	C.
19	9 thin, yeasty movements. Flatulence and dizziness began to pass away after the morning stool.	11 thin, yeasty stools. After breakfast began to feel better and improved all day.	9 thin, yeasty stools, after which dizziness subsided and felt quite cheerful by evening.
20	3 stools moderately thin. Numbness passing off. Head clearer. Feels quite well.	4 stools, thin and yeasty. Feeling quite well and improved all day.	3 stools moderately thin. Rapidly improving.
21	2 stools of fair consistence, and feels quite well.	3 stools. Feels well and gaining all day.	2 stools; feels well and gaining rapidly.
22	1 stool. Feels well and unusually bright.	2 stools of fair consistence, and feels well.	1 healthy stool. Feels perfectly well.

DAY.	D.	E.	F.
19	11 thin, yeasty stools during the morning, after which began to improve and felt quite well by night.	10 thin, yeasty stools before 10 A. M., after which improved rapidly, and at night felt well.	11 thin, yeasty stools. After breakfast began to improve fast. Greatly better by evening.
20	4 stools moderately thin. Numbness disappearing. Dizziness going fast.	4 stools. Feels well and gaining rapidly.	5 thin stools. Feels well and improving rapidly in all respects.
21	2 stools. Gaining rapidly. Feels well and clear headed.	1 stool. Feels well and gaining rapidly.	2 stools. Cheerful. Feels well and gaining fast.
22	1 good, hard, healthy stool. Feels well and happy.	1 healthy stool. Feels well and clear headed.	1 stool. Feels unusually well and cheerful.

My boarders, on the 19th morning, all presented such a forlorn, dilapidated appearance, that I feared I should lose my reputation as a caterer, and also all my guests, unless I changed my diet list. They had all lost heavily in weight, and were much debilitated.

A weighed 138 lbs.	Loss in 18 days	22 lbs.
B " 116 "	" "	29 "
C " 136 "	" "	19 "
D " 143 "	" "	23 "
E " 147 "	" "	25 "
F " 126 "	" "	22 "

When on the morning of the 19th day, I set before them nice beefsteaks, freed from fat and white tissue, they were all greatly delighted and ate ravenously of them. I gave to each 10 ounces of meat, with a good cup of clear coffee. Beef seasoned with butter, pepper and salt; no other food or drinks. At dinner gave each 12 ounces of beefsteak, prepared as for breakfast, and half a pint of clear tea. The meal was hugely enjoyed.

All now began to breathe easier and to feel clearer about the head. Passages less frequent, though still large and numerous. During the afternoon, all were in a state of enjoyable relief, and were ready to speak a good word for their host and his house.

At supper, gave each 10 ounces of beefsteak, with a cup of

clear tea. The meal was greatly relished. The evening was a pleasant one, all having a sense of relief from the extreme flatulence, bewildered heads, oppressed breathing and numbness of previous days. Retired at 9 p. m. All slept soundly and were ready to rise at 6 a. m. on the 20th morning. For breakfast, gave to each 12 ounces of broiled steak and half a pint of clear coffee. Passages from bowels greatly lessened in quantity and frequency. Bloating almost gone. Heads quite clear, and all cheerful and happy. At dinner, gave each 1 lb. of nice broiled steak and half a pint of clear tea: meal greatly relished. All felt well and began to lose their haggard, shrunken look. Circulation good; heads clear; bloating gone; movements beginning to be quite natural and few in number. At supper gave to each 12 ounces of broiled steak and half a pint of clear tea. All felt well during the evening. Retired at 9 p. m. Slept soundly.

Called up on 21st day at 6 a. m. All feeling well and anxious for breakfast. Gave each 1 lb. of broiled steak and half a slice of bread, with half a pint of clear coffee. All enjoyed the breakfast. Half an hour after breakfast gave them a brisk walk of two miles. All well, and felt better, brighter and clearer than before the experiments began. Bloating, diarrhœa, ringing in ears and dizzy head all gone. At dinner gave to each 1 lb. beefsteak, 1 slice of bread and half a pint of clear tea. No diarrhœa; stools quite natural except more profuse. At supper gave each 14 ounces of broiled steak, half a slice of bread, and half a pint of clear tea. Meal greatly enjoyed. All gaining rapidly in strength and feeling splendidly. Retired at 9 p. m. All slept soundly.

Called up on 22d morning at 6 a. m. All in good trim, and loud in their praise of their host and his table. Gave each 1 lb. of broiled steak, half a pint of clear coffee and a slice of bread and butter. The meal was much enjoyed. All felt unusually well, clear headed and happy. Half an hour after breakfast gave them a long walk. At 12 m. each had 1 lb. of broiled steak, a slice of bread and a cup of clear coffee, which they took with great relish.

After finishing the meal, I paid off my boarders and discharged them. With a feeling of regret and reluctance (I think on both sides) we separated. Still, they could not realize how I could keep up and "make both ends meet," while running a boarding house on this plan. I may add that I had throughout shared their diet, discipline and experiences in all respects.

L.

EXPERIMENTS IN FEEDING ON OATMEAL CONTINUOUSLY, AS AN EXCLUSIVE DIET.

In October, 1857, I placed four hearty, well men upon oatmeal porridge as an exclusive diet. It was seasoned with butter, pepper and salt. Cold water was drank between meals, and a pint of coffee, seasoned with sugar and milk, was taken at each meal. The men were the most healthy and vigorous I could procure. All regarded themselves as perfectly well, and none had ever suffered any severe illness. Their ages ranged from twenty-three to thirty-eight years. I required them all to live with me continually, night and day, and to take no food or drinks other than what I gave them. They were to receive $30 per month each, with board and lodging. I subjected myself to the same rules and regulations, asking of them nothing but what I would and did do myself. This gave them a confidence and pride in the work, each striving to outdo the other in the strict observance of the rules.

At noon on the 9th of October, the rigid diet began. The noon and night meals of the first day were greatly enjoyed by all. Retired at 9 p. m. and slept soundly and well. All were called up at 6 a. m. next morning. Meals were taken at 7 a. m., 12 m. and 6 p. m. On the afternoon of the second day, all began to be more or less flatulent. Bowels bloated, and wind in motion in the large bowels. Each had a constipated movement of the bowels during the middle and latter part of the day, accompanied by much wind. Before the exclusive oatmeal diet began, each had one regular movement of the bowels every morning.

At 4 p. m. gave the men a walk of about two miles, which helped to work off the flatulence. All retired at 9 p. m. and slept soundly.

At 6 a. m. of the third day, all were called and required to take a cold sponge bath. Before the bath, a dull, heavy feeling pervaded the entire party; this was partially relieved by the bath. Very flatulent; bowels more or less distended and uncomfortable. Ate quite heartily at the 7 a. m. breakfast, each drinking the pint of coffee allowed.

At 8 a. m. walked the men out for about two miles. This somewhat cleared away the dullness, and worked off the flatus. There was a general feeling of thirst during the forenoon, which was satisfied by a free indulgence in cold water.

Dined at 12 m. At 2 p. m. all were feeling quite bloated and very uncomfortable. Gave them a two mile walk, which to some extent relieved the distended, dull feelings. Not one had a passage of the bowels on the third day. Appetites still good, but not ravenous, as on the first day. Retired at 9 p. m. A stupid, heavy feeling pervaded the household. Very flatulent, with colic pains.

The fourth day, all rather dull and quite flatulent, with occasional colic pains. All had movements of the bowels in the latter part of the day, accompanied by much wind. Appetites good.

The fifth day found all about the same as on the fourth day, except that the symptoms were aggravated. Each had a small, constipated movement in latter part of the day and evening.

The sixth day, all the derangements of the fifth day were more pronounced. Each had a small, difficult movement during the latter part of the day and evening. Very flatulent.

The seventh day, the derangements of the sixth day were still more marked. Flatulence and constipation increasing. Each had a very small, hard movement during the latter part of the day and evening.

I will indicate the boarders by the letters A, B, C and D. They exercised daily. Morning and evening walk of two miles. Rising hour, 6 a. m. Retiring hour, 9 p. m.

The following table will show their symptoms under the diet named, from the 8th to the 34th day, inclusive : —

DAY.	A.	B.	C.	D.
8	Very flatulent. Wandering pains in bowels. Head dull and achy. Constipated. Appetite fair but not ravenous. Had a constipated small movement at 3 p. m.	Very flatulent. Constant rumbling in bowels with some pain. Head aching and slightly dizzy. Singing in ears on retiring. Constipated, small movement at 1.30 p. m. accompanied by much wind.	Bowels much distended with gas and some colic pains. Very dull and head aches. Bowels constipated, moving scantily at 4.30 p. m. accompanied by much wind. Appetite fair. Is slightly feverish and thirsty.	Very flatulent. Pains in stomach and bowels. Ears ring. Head aches and is slightly constipated. Bowels bewildered. No movement.
9	Stomach and bowels full of wind in motion. Wandering pains. Head mixed and aches. Ringing in ears. Constipated. Appetite good. Thirsty. Had small, constipated movement at 5 p. m. Feces hard, dry, light-colored, and rather sticky. Feet prickle.	Stomach and bowels distended with wind in motion. Colic pains. Head dizzy and achy. Constipated. Had small, difficult movement at 4.30 p. m. Feces light in color. Singing in ears.	Very flatulent. Bowels sore as if bruised. Colic pains. Head mixed and achy. Had a small, hard movement of the bowels at 8 p. m. Feverish and thirsty. Appetite good.	Stomach and bowels much distended with gas and full of wandering pains. Singing in ears. Head mixed and achy. Had a hard, scanty movement at 11 a. m. accompanied with wind. Feet prickle.
10	Stomach and bowels much distended with gas; full of wandering pains. Bowels lame as if bruised. Very dull and stupid on rising. Head mixed and achy. Constipated. No movement. Ears ring. Appetite fair. Feet and fingers prickle. Heart palpitates on much exertion.	Dull and stupid on rising. Bowels and stomach much distended with gas. Head mixed and ears ring. Bowels constipated. No movement. Pain in small of back. Feet prickle. Appetite quite good. Heart palpitates from any over-exertion.	Very dumpish and tired. Bowels and stomach greatly distended with gas and full of wandering pains. Abdomen lame as if bruised. Ears ring. Head mixed and achy. Feet prickle. Heart palpitates on over-exertion. Small, constipated movement with much wind at 8.30 p. m.	Dull and tired all day. Stomach and bowels much bloated and hard; full of wandering pains. Pain in back. Feet and hands prickle. Head mixed and achy. Ears ring. Heart palpitates on much exertion. No movement of bowels.
11	On rising, very dull and mixed, with dizzy head. Pains in temples and occiput. Ears ring. Heart palpitates on exertion. Constipated. Bowels very much bloated. Colic pains. Feet prickle. A small difficult movement of hardened feces at 3.30 p. m. accompanied with much wind. Appetite fair. Bruised, lamed feeling over bowels. Lumbar pains.	Stupid and dull. Head mixed and aches. Ears ring. Hands and feet prickle. Bowels much disturbed with wind and full of little colic pains. Pain in small of back. Appetite fairly good. Feverish and thirsty. Heart palpitates on over-exertion. Small, hard movement at 4 p. m. with much wind. Lame in umbilical region as if bruised.	Very dull on rising. Felt better after his bath. Bowels greatly disturbed with wind and full of wandering pains. Bowels feel lame. Ears ring. Head mixed and achy. Feet and hands prickle. Heart palpitates on over-exertion; breathing oppressed when walking fast. Pains between shoulders and in small of back. No movement. Appetite fair. Thirsty and feverish.	Very tired and dull all day. Bowels greatly distended with gas, and full of aches; feel lame as if bruised. Heart palpitates on exertion. Breathing becomes short and hurried. Hands and feet prickle. Ears ring. Head dizzy and mixed. Memory poor. Disinclined to exertion. Small constipated movement at 8 p. m. with much wind. Feverish and thirsty. Pains in back.

DAY.	A.	B.	C.	D.
12	Stomach and bowels very much bloated and full of wandering pains. Neuralgic pains in heart. Oppressed breathing on over-exertion. Head mixed and achy. Prickling sensation in limbs. Pains in small of back. Very constipated. No movement. Feverish, thirsty. Singing in ears. Forgetful. Languid and disposed to lie down. Feet cold. Appetite fairly good.	Greatly disturbed with wind. Colic frequently. Very dull and easily exhausted on exertion. Disposed to lie down. Head confused. Ringing in ears. Feet and hands prickle. Heart weak and beats irregularly. Sitting pulse 66 to the minute. Very constipated. Back weak. Feverish and thirsty. Appetite fair. Disturbed with acid eructations.	Very tired and languid. Did not want to get up. Felt better after sponge bath. Singing in ears. Head mixed and confused. Pains in back of head and temples. Heart intermits, losing every 4th or 5th beat. Sitting pulse, 62 to the minute. Ate quite heartily. Very bloated and full of wandering pains. Oppressed for breath on over-exertion. Acid eructations. No movement.	Awoke with severe headache. Acid eructations. Stomach and bowels disturbed with flatus. Appetite good but eats mechanically. Don't know when he has enough. Head dizzy. Quite forgetful. Ears ring. Thinks he is getting crazy. Heart palpitates on severe exertions. Loses every 3d or 4th beat: 58 to minute. No movement. Feet and hands partially numb. Pain in small of back.
13	Nightmare during night. Heart irregular in its beat, about 60 to minute sitting. Head mixed and confused. Forgetful. Stomach and bowels greatly distended with gas. Colic pains. Head full and achy. No movement. Feet and hands prickle. Ears ring. Pains in small of back. Breathing oppressed when exercising much. Appetite fair. Thirsty and feverish. Thinks he is losing his mind.	Sleep disturbed with frightful dreams. Very tired and wants to lie down. Stomach and bowels much distended with gas and full of colic pains. Heart beat irregular and 59 to the minute, sitting. Head mixed, dizzy and aching. Ears ring. No movement. Appetite fairly good. Feet and hands prickle, and feel heavy. Feverish and thirsty. A choking feeling in swallowing.	Had a heavy, dead sleep and awoke very tired. Did not want to get up. After a sponge bath felt better. Head mixed. Ears ring. Feet and hands prickle. Feels heavy and full. Forgetful. Heart beats irregularly and 62 to the minute; palpitates on exertion. No movement. Very much distended with gas and full of colic pains. Appetite is fair.	Disturbed in sleep by bad dreams. Stomach and bowels much distended with gas. Ears ring. Head mixed and dizzy. Forgetful. Thinks he is getting crazy. No movement. Feet and hands numb. Heart irregular; 58 to the minute. Breathing oppressed on exertion. Appetite fair. A choking feeling on swallowing.
14	Sleep heavy and with bad dreams. Awoke dull and mixed. Felt better after sponge bath. Bowels and stomach painfully distended with gas. Very constipated. Scanty, hard movement late in day with much gas. Pains in back and limbs. Head bewildered and aching. Feet and hands prickle. Heart palpitates on exertion. Ears ring. Mouth and throat covered with sticky mucus. Feverish and thirsty. Appetite still fair. Pulse irregular and 59 to the minute.	Sleep disturbed with nightmare. Very tired on rising. Better after sponge bath. Head mixed, confused and achy. Forgetful. Ears ring. Feet and hands prickle and feel numb and heavy. Back aches. Stomach and bowels greatly distended with gas, and aching. Abdomen feels lame as if bruised. Reels in walking. Breathing oppressed on exertion. Thirsty. Raises thick, sticky mucus. Appetite fair. No movement. Pulse irregular and 58 to the minute.	Wakeful all night. Tired and dull on rising. Felt better after bath and breakfast. Head mixed and confused all day. Ears ring. Feet and hands prickle and feet swollen and heavy. Stomach and bowels greatly disturbed with gas and full of colic pains. Abdomen lame as if bruised. Unsteady in walking. Heart palpitates on over-exertion. Pulse 57 to the minute and irregular. Breathing short, oppressed on over - exertion. Scanty movement at 3 p. m. with much flatus. Appetite fair.	Sleep disturbed by troubled dreams. Awoke feeling dull and tired. Head achy and mixed. Unsteady in walking. Ears ring. Bowels and stomach greatly distended with gas and full of little pains. Abdomen lame as if bruised. Pulse irregular and 58 to the minute. Heart palpitates on over-exertion and breathing oppressed. Scanty, hard movement of bowels at 7 p. m. accompanied with much wind. Back aches. Feet and hands prickle and feel numb. Appetite fair.
15	Nightmare and bad dreams. Very dull, mixed and stupid on rising. Felt better after bath and breakfast. Very flatulent; stomach and bowels much distended with gas. Full of colic pains. Abdomen lame as if bruised. Ears ring. 56 pulsations per minute. Feet and hands prickle and feel numb. Mouth and throat covered with sticky mucus. Thirst. No movement. Appetite is fair.	Wakeful and nervous all night. Very flatulent and full of small colic pains. Small, hard movement of the bowels soon after rising. Head dizzy and mixed. Forgetful. Feet and hands are prickly and numb. Legs seem heavy and not under perfect control. Ears ring. Mouth and throat covered with sticky mucus. Pulse irregular and 58 to the minute. Appetite fair.	Sleep disturbed with bad dreams. Dull and stupid on rising, but somewhat improved by bath and breakfast. Heart palpitates on exertion and misses every 5th or 6th beat. Legs and arms prickle and feel numb and heavy. Feet cold. Unsteady in walking. Abdomen lame as if bruised. No movement. Painfully distended with gas. Appetite only fair. Thirsty.	Sleep disturbed by unpleasant dreams. Dull and mixed on rising. A little better after bath and breakfast. Bowels and stomach greatly disturbed with gas. Abdomen feels lame and bruised. No movement. Pulse irregular, 58 to the minute. Any over - exertion causes oppressed breathing and palpitation. Appetite fair, but eats without much relish.

DAY.	A.	B.	C.	D.
16 to 24 inclusive	Sleep much disturbed with bad dreams. Bowels and stomach painfully distended with wind and abdomen lame as if bruised. Continued constipation. One scanty, hard movement on the 18th inst.; one on 22d inst. and a loose movement on 23d and 24th. Head gradually growing more and more mixed and confused. Heart more irregular in beat and increased palpitation on exertion, with oppressed breathing. Ears ring. Eyes blur in reading. Throat and fauces dry and sticky. Limbs prickle much and are heavy, and drag in walking. Pains in back and head. Appetite moderate. At times a choking feeling in swallowing. Submaxillary glands tender and somewhat swollen. Feels "as if his mind was giving way."	Nights greatly disturbed with wakefulness and nightmare. Has frightful dreams. Stomach and bowels greatly distended with gas, which he is unable to eructate or pass. Full of colic pains. A feeling of numbness and weight in limbs. Head mixed, dizzy and at times numb. Ears ring. Eyesight growing dim. Throat and mouth covered with sticky mucus. Heart beats irregular, and breathing oppressed on exertion. Had a hard, scanty movement on 19th, 20th, and 21st inst. and a full movement 22d and 23d inst., accompanied by considerable wind. Neuralgic pains in left arm and leg, and small of back. Abdomen very lame as if bruised. Swelling of feet towards evening. Very thirsty much of time. Appetite fair.	Feels languid, tired and depressed most of time. Sleep much disturbed by frightful dreams. Sometimes sees double, and imagines he sees snakes, devils, etc. Talks in sleep; often wakes in fright when heart palpitates violently. Head mixed, confused and dizzy. Forgetful. Bowels and stomach greatly distended with gas and filled with wandering pains. Neuralgic pains in left arm, side and leg, with numbness in extremities. Legs feel heavy and has lost perfect control over them. A small, constipated movement on 18th and 23d inst. with much wind. Loose on 24th. Thirsty much of time. Throat, fauces, and mouth sticky. Heart palpitates on exertion; breathing oppressed. Abdomen lame. Choking feeling often in swallowing.	Very tired and languid nearly all the time. Stomach and bowels painfully distended with gas. Wakeful nights; when sleeping has frightful dreams. Abdomen lame as if bruised. A small, constipated movement on 18th and 23d. Head mixed, confused, and dizzy. Unsteady in walking. Not very good use of legs; they feel heavy and numb. After the 20th feet begin to swell toward evening. Heart palpitates on much exertion; breathing becomes oppressed and short. Neuralgic pains in heart, left arm, back, and left leg. After the 22d the glands of neck become tender and somewhat swollen. Appetite fair.
25 and 26	All the symptoms and conditions of the 24th are aggravated. On the morning of 25th had 2 large, full, yeasty movements, with much flatus; after this experienced some relief from distention and oppressed breathing. On morning of 26th had 3 large, thin, yeasty movements, accompanied by much wind, and followed by relief. Pains in lumbar region. Legs and feet heavy, clumsy and numb. Ears ring and much confused. Quite deaf at times; memory poor. Dizzy. Heart palpitates on the least exertion.	Bad night; full of colic pains; slept but little. At 6 a. m. had a profuse movement; another at 7.30 a. m. with much wind, after which felt better. On 26th had 3 movements before 9 a. m. all large, thin, and yeasty. Felt much brighter afterward. Legs and feet numb and heavy. Pains in small of back, running down into thighs. Extremities cold and clammy. Head dizzy and confused. Ears ring; hearing obtuse. Urine scanty and high colored. Heart palpitates on exertion, its beats are irregular. Feels dull, tired, drowsy, and disinclined to move. Thirsty and feverish.	Slept fairly well. Towards morning of 25th was awakened with severe colic pains and at 5.30 a. m. had a profuse, watery, yeasty movement, and another about one hour after. Both were accompanied by a large quantity of wind; felt greatly relieved after. On morning of 26th had 2 large, thin, yeasty movements before 6 a. m. and a 3d at 8 a. m., both preceded by colic pains. Passed much confused and dizzy; memory poor. Ears ring; hearing obtuse. Pains in legs and back. Lower extremities numb. Reels in walking. Soles feel like cushions. Thirsty and feverish.	Sleep disturbed by troubled dreams. At 7.30 a. m. had very large, thin, yeasty movement, with much flatus, and preceded by colic pains. Before 9 a. m. on 26th had 3 large, yeasty movements with much wind, and severe colic pains before the movements. Head mixed, confused and dizzy. Ears ring. Memory poor. Very dull and stupid. Legs and feet numb and clumsy. Lumbar pains. Urine scanty, high colored, and deposits heavy sediment of urates on cooling. Feels tired and does not like to be disturbed. Appetite fair. Thirsty and somewhat feverish.
27	Sleep disturbed with bad dreams. Colic pains toward morning. 3 profuse, thin, yeasty movements before 9 a. m. with much wind. After this felt better. Growing more confused and dizzy. Ears ring. Legs and feet numb, heavy and unable to use them well. Appetite fair. Dull, tired and stupid. Tongue thick. Voice weak and husky. Eyes look a little wild.	Slept fairly well till awakened at 4 a. m. with colic pains. At 5 a. m. had profuse, yeasty movement, with much flatus. Before 10 a. m. had 2 more equally large and windy passages, then felt better. Head dizzy, mixed, confused. Eyes wild and staring. Ears ring. Hearing impaired. Legs and feet numb and cushioned soles. Voice husky and weak. Fauces and mouth covered with sticky mucus. Thirsty, feverish.	Restless and filled with little colic pains. Had 4 large, thin, yeasty movements, with much flatus, before 10 a. m. Head confused and dizzy. Ears ring. Eyes water. Mouth and fauces covered with sticky mucus. Legs and feet numb and unwieldy. Back aches and has shooting sciatic pains. Voice weak; is disinclined to talk or move about. Appetite fair.	Uncomfortable night from colic pains. At 4 a. m. had a large, thin, yeasty movement, accompanied by much wind. Before 11 a. m. had three more similar movements. Head dizzy and confused. Eyes watery. Ears ring; hearing impaired. Mouth and fauces covered with sticky mucus. Legs and feet numb and clumsy. Pains in back and thighs.

DAY.	A.	B.	C.	D.
28	All the symptoms and conditions of the 27th intensified. Had 4 profuse, watery, yeasty movements before 11 a. m. accompanied by a large amount of gas. Feels weak. Legs numb and very clumsy to handle.	Had 5 very profuse yeasty movements of the bowels before 11.30 a. m. accompanied by a great amount of gas. All the other symptoms and conditions of the 27th are aggravated.	Had 5 profuse yeasty thin movements accompanied by much gas, before 10 a. m. All the other symptoms and conditions of the 27th intensified.	Had 6 profuse, thin, and yeasty movements before noon; passed a great deal of gas. Other symptoms and conditions of 27th aggravated.
29	Had 7 profuse movements of the bowels before noon. Passages very thin and yeasty accompanied by a great amount of gas.	6 profuse, thin, watery movements before 1 p. m. Feels very weak, and large discharge of gas.	Had 8 profuse, thin, yeasty movements before 1 p. m. Feels very weak and prickles all over. Heart palpitates, is irregular and 45 to 48 per minute.	Had 7 profuse, thin, and yeasty passages before 10 a. m. Very weak and feels numb all over. Quite deaf and listless.

All the other symptoms and conditions of the 27th aggravated.

30	All had a very uncomfortable night. No good rest. A had 9 movements of the bowels before noon. B 8. C 11. D 10. The movements were all profuse, thin and yeasty, accompanied by much flatus. Other symptoms and conditions of the 27th all intensified. Concluded it was neither prudent nor safe to carry the experiment any further. So at noon gave all a nice beefsteak and cup of clear coffee, which were greatly enjoyed. At 4 p. m. gave each man a dessert spoonful of Rochelle salts in a goblet of water. This gave from 2 to 3 vigorous and profuse movements of the bowels, in each case before 6 p. m. and cleaned out the yeasty matters pretty effectually. At 6.30 p. m. gave each a good meal of broiled beefsteak and a cup of clear coffee. All ate with a relish and felt greatly improved in every way. Retired at 9 p. m. A very comfortable and restful night for all.			
31	All felt quite well after a fair night's rest. Partook of a good breakfast of broiled beefsteak and clear tea. The two following meals were the same. A had 4 movements of the bowels during the day, all in the forenoon and much smaller than the movements yesterday. B had 3 movements, rather profuse. C had 4 large and 1 small movement. D had 4 movements. The day passed pleasantly and enjoyably.			
32	All up at 6 a. m. feeling quite well after a good night's rest. All three meals — breakfast, dinner, and supper — were of broiled beefsteak and a cup of clear tea. A had 3 movements during the day, rather profuse. B had 2 large and 1 small movement. C had 3 movements. D had 2 profuse movements and 1 small one. The movements all occurred during the morning and forenoon. The dizziness, numbness, unsteady gait and ringing in ears all disappearing rapidly.			
33	At 6 a. m. all were up and in the best of spirits. Diet same as on the 32d. A had 2 movements. B had 2 movements, 1 large and 1 small one. C had 3 movements, 1 large and 2 small. D had 3 movements, 1 large and 2 small. All the symptoms and conditions improving fast.			
34	All up at 6 a. m. feeling quite well. Gait steady. Numbness and ringing in ears gone. Heads clear. A happy "crowd," full of the best of humor. Diet and drinks same as yesterday. A had but 1 movement, which was quite natural. B had 1 large and 1 small movement. C had 2 moderate movements, and D 2 quite free operations. After supper all were so well and happy that I paid them off and let them go to their respective homes.			

LI.

EXPERIMENTS CONNECTED WITH PRODUCING CONSUMPTION OF
THE BOWELS, OR CHRONIC DIARRHŒA OF ARMIES, BY FEED-
ING UPON ARMY BISCUIT.

IT was found that whenever soldiers were thrown largely
upon the use of hard bread, or army biscuit, as a diet, a peculiar train of abnormal manifestations presented themselves.
These are : —

1. Constipation.

2. This constipation is preceded, accompanied and followed
by fermentative changes and the development of intestinal
gases and yeast plants (Saccharomyces and Mycoderma) in the
food in the stomach and intestines.

3. These fermentative changes are always worse towards
evening and during the night, and go on increasing from day
to day till : —

4. Finally the gases and yeast plants and other products of
fermentation developed, produce so much irritation, commotion,
distention and paralysis of the intestinal walls, that diarrhœa
ensues, which soon becomes chronic, and is not at all amenable
to the treatment of ordinary diarrhœal conditions.

5. Accompanying the fermentative changes is always a paralytic tendency, more or less strongly marked. This is manifested
in the alimentary canal, and especially in the larger intestines;
next in the extremities, the legs prickling and " getting asleep,"
frequently, with ringing in the ears and a numb, mixed up or
confused feeling in the head, etc. These are manifestations
pertaining to the history of the disease known as Locomotor
Ataxy.

6. A cough, accompanied by more or less hoarseness, usually sets in, especially during the night and on rising in the morning. It is also accompanied by the expectoration of a thick, cream-colored, sweetish mucus.

7. This is followed by more or less constriction in breathing with frequently palpitation of the heart on any excitement.

8. After the diarrhœa sets in, there is generally a remarkable tendency to fibrinous depositions in the heart (Thrombosis), and to the clogging up of the pulmonary vessels with fibrinous clots (Embolism), with pains and aches in extremities and back.

9. The diarrhœa is not so likely to come on when the men are actively engaged, as it is when they go into camp and are less active.

The active exercise seems to aid in working the starchy food out of the stomach into the bowels, where it is digested before it gets to fermenting badly.

To demonstrate more positively that these abnormal conditions had their origin in the too exclusive use of Army biscuit as a food, it was determined to institute a series of experiments upon the exclusive use of this kind of food, as tried upon strong, healthy men, in a healthy locality, and free from the enfeebling influences of Army life. Accordingly, on arriving at Cincinnati, Ohio, I engaged the services of three strong, vigorous men of good habits and in the prime of life, for this purpose.

The experiments were conducted with watchful care from day to day, and the results were most convincing and conclusive in favor of the previous observations made upon the soldiers, as will be seen from the following daily records of the experiments.

October 12th, at noon, began feeding the men exclusively upon Army biscuit. For drink used water, to which at dinner and tea about one ounce of good whiskey was added. Gave the men the whiskey, as they were used to taking about two or three drinks daily.

Hours for Meals: 7 a. m., 12 m., and 5 p. m.

Date. Oct. 12th, 1863.	Mr. H., aged 36. Weight, 150 lbs. Height, 5 ft. 10 in.	Mr. B., Age 40. Weight, 158 lbs. Height, 5 ft. 9½ in.	Mr. S., Age 38. Weight, 152 lbs. Height, 5 ft. 9 in.
Oct. 12th, noon.	Relished the new diet and ate heartily. Slept well at night.	Ate heartily of the new diet. Slept well.	Ate moderately of the new diet. Slept well.
13th.	Passage from the bowels at his usual time, but less free than normal. Was accustomed to have a free stool every morning. Felt well during 13th, eating heartily and sleeping well at night.	One passage from bowels at 8 a. m. Accustomed to having a passage every morning. Ate with a good appetite; was very thirsty and drank freely of cold water. Slept well.	One constipated passage at 10 a. m. Accustomed to having a passage every morning before breakfast. Ate ravenously. Thirsty during afternoon and evening. Drank water. Slept well.
14th.	Constipated, having no passage from bowels, although repaired to the water closet as usual. Felt well during the day and night.	Had a constipated passage at 3 p. m., previous to which was very much bloated. Ate well. Very thirsty. Drank freely of water. A little dizziness or mixed confused feeling. Slept well.	No movement of bowels. Very much bloated, with considerable uneasiness. Mixed and confused. Ate heartily. Thirsty, and drank freely of water. Slept well.
15th.	In the morning had a difficult, scant passage of pale, plastic feces. Full of flatus. During the day had occasionally slight dizziness and less muscular vigor than usual. Slept well during the night.	No passage of the bowels to-day. Much bloated. The flatus in constant motion, producing much uneasiness. Mixed and dizzy. Has a feeling of lassitude. Slept well.	Had a scant, constipated passage of pale plastic feces at 5 p. m. Very flatulent, with considerable uneasiness in bowels. Mixed and confused. Feels dull, not much inclined to move. Slept soundly.
16th.	Had no stool. Considerable flatus and rumbling in bowels. During the evening ate a couple of apples. Slept well during the night.	No movement. Much bloated. Feels very uneasy in bowels. Quite mixed and confused. Prickling in feet and hands. Ate an apple after supper. Slept well, retiring at 9 p. m.	No movement. Very flatulent, with colic pains and much rumbling in bowels. Feels dull and stupid. Ate an apple after supper. Slept well.
17th.	Had a very scant passage of pale, plastic feces about 8 a. m. After passage had a throbbing and heat in the lower portion of large intestines. Towards and during the evening considerable flatus, with some eructations. Before retiring ate an apple and drank freely of water. Slept well.	Scant movement of pale plastic feces at 1 p. m., accompanied by much wind. Felt better. A burning and throbbing in rectum after passage. Has creeping chills and feels confused and mixed. Ate an apple before retiring. Very flatulent and uneasy. Restless sleep, troubled dreams.	No movement. Very much bloated. Feels mixed, confused, dull and stupid. Hands and feet prickle. Very thirsty; drank freely of water. Ate an apple after supper. Slept uneasily, with troubled dreams.
18th.	Had no passage. Mixed and dizzy all day with considerable muscular debility. Appetite excellent. Still relishes the food, but would like it better if he had some meat with it. Lower bowels feel numb, distended and torpid. Full of flatus during evening and night. Slept well.	No movement. Very much bloated with much uneasiness in bowels. Head mixed and confused. Hands and feet prickle. Feels languid and disinclined to move. Ate well and slept well.	Had a scant passage at 10 a. m. of pale sticky feces. After passage had a throbbing and heat in lower bowels. Very flatulent in afternoon and evening, with much uneasiness. Mixed and confused. Hands and feet prickle; head feels numb. Sleep uneasy: dreaming.
19th.	No passage. Felt a mixed, confused dizziness all day with want of muscular vigor. Exercised freely in walking and felt better. Slept well during the night.	No movement. Very much bloated and oppressed at times in breathing. Heart flutters on any severe exertion. Feels weak. Head mixed and dizzy. Feet and hands prickle. Sleep uneasy. Troubled dreams.	No movement. Very flatulent with much rumbling in bowels. Wind in constant motion. Very uncomfortable. Head mixed and confused. Feet and hands prickle. Sleep disturbed with dreams.

DAY.	MR. H.	MR. B.	MR. S.
20th.	Had a difficult, scant passage of pale, plastic feces, after which had a heat and throbbing in the lower bowels, which were inactive and partially paralyzed. During the evening and night much distended with flatus, with eructations and passages of wind. Slept well.	Had a scant passage at 4 p. m. of pale, sticky feces, accompanied by much flatus. After which throbbing and heat in lower bowels. Head mixed and confused. Feels as if he were "getting crazy." Feet and hands prickle. Greatly distended with wind during afternoon and night. Sleep uneasy.	No movement. Bowels greatly disturbed with wind. Head mixed and confused. Very languid. Ate well and drank freely of cold water to quench thirst. Feet and hands prickle. Sleep uneasy with troubled dreams.
21st.	No passage. Much disturbed with flatus. Mixed and dizzy all day. Prickling in feet and hands.	No movement. Very flatulent. Mixed, confused and dizzy. Feet and hands prickle. Sleep is uneasy.	A scant movement of pale, putty-like feces. Heat and throbbing after, in lower bowels. Dizzy and mixed. Ate well. Slept soundly.
22d.	Yesterday and to-day has had a numb, dizzy feeling in the head, which is partially dissipated by walking vigorously. Appetite good. Feet and legs prickle and feel heavy, and not under the best control. Pain in small of back.	No movement. Very much bloated and uneasy in bowels, which was partially relieved by walking. Head mixed, confused and dizzy. Dull and stupid. Slept quite well, but dreamed and talked in sleep. Legs and feet feel heavy and numb.	No movement. Very much distended with flatus. Mixed and confused. Hands and feet prickle ; head feels numb. Ate well. Sleep troubled with dreams. Legs feel numb and heavy, and he trips in walking.
23d.	Had a difficult, scant passage of pale, putty-like plastic feces. Lower bowels more inactive than usual. Passed considerable wind. During evening and night troubled much with rumbling and disturbance of bowels with flatus. Legs and feet numb : walks clumsily. Pains in small of back. Slept well.	A small constipated movement of pale, putty-like feces, accompanied by much wind. Numb feeling in lower bowels and prickling in feet and hands. Head mixed and confused. A swimming sensation on lying down. Troubled with great distension of bowels, noon, evening and night, from flatus. Sleep disturbed.	No movement. Much distended with flatus in constant motion. Head mixed and confused. Feet and hands prickle. Heart palpitates on any exertion. Pulse intermits, closing 1 beat every 4 to 6. Ate quite well. Sleep disturbed with troubled dreams. Legs feel heavy and numb. Drags the feet in walking.
24th.	No passage. Felt well, but not strong as usual. Head feels numb, legs often "go to sleep." During evening and night the bowels distended much with wind which appears in constant motion. Legs and feet numb and heavy. Has a shuffling walk. Soles of feet seem to be cushioned.	No movement. Head dizzy, mixed, confused; numb. Hands and feet prickle. Numb feeling in bowels. Heart palpitates on much exertion. Bowels painfully distended with flatus. Sleep uneasy. Legs and feet numb and not under good control. Stumbles readily in walking. Pain and weakness in small of back.	Scant, constipated movement at 4 p. m. of pale, ash-colored, putty-like feces. Throbbing and heat in lower bowels. Painfully bloated during evening and night. Head numb, mixed and confused. Feet and hands prickle. Legs and feet numb and heavy. Losing control over them. Soles feel as if cushioned.
25th.	Had no passage; no pains. Less vigorous than usual. Peculiar dead numbness about the head. Appetite good. Upper bowels and stomach distended with flatus in motion during the evening and night. Ate 2 apples before retiring. Walked about 2 miles. Feet and legs numb and heavy. Drags the feet in walking. Wakeful.	No movement. Bowels greatly distended with flatus, which gives much uneasiness. Head numb, mixed and confused ; swims around on lying down. Heart palpitates on exertion. Ate well. Pain in small of back. Legs and feet numb and heavy. Walks with shuffling gait. Soles seem to be cushioned. Sleep uneasy.	No movement. Bowels greatly distended with flatus. Head mixed, numb, confused. Heart palpitates on exertion. Feet and hands "get asleep." Swimming sensations on lying down. Ate well. Sciatic pains. Legs and feet numb and heavy. Reels in walking. Soles feel as if cushioned. Sleep disturbed ; troubled dreams.

DAY.	MR. H.	MR. B.	MR. S.
26th.	Had difficult, scant passage of pale, putty-like, ash-colored feces. Felt passably well, with the exception of weakness and numb sensations in head, legs and lower bowels. Appetite good. Tongue clean. Very eager for meat. Bowels much distended with flatus during evening and night, on account of which sleep was much disturbed. Feet and legs same as on 25th inst.	No movement. Head feels numb and much confused. Feet and hands prickle, feel numb and heavy. Bowels painfully bloated with flatus without having the ability to eructate or pass it. Tongue clean. Very thirsty; drank freely of cold water. Heart palpitates on exertion, with some irregularity in beats. Ate well. Sleep disturbed by the uneasy bowels.	No movement. Head feels numb and mixed, with a swimming sensation on lying down. Bowels painfully distended with flatus: unable to eructate or pass it. Considerable thirst: flashes of heat followed by chilly feelings. Heart palpitates on exertion; some irregularity in beats. Ate well. Sleep disturbed by wandering thoughts and troubled dreams.
27th.	Had no passage. Felt a heat and throbbing in the lower intestines. Appetite good. Less vigorous. Wakeful during night. Disturbed with flatus and dizzy, mixed sensations. No change for the better in feet and legs.	At 1 p. m. had a small, plastic, pale, putty-like passage, followed by heat and throbbing in the lower bowels. Lower bowels and head feel numb. Head confused. Swims on lying down. Feet and hands prickle and feel numb. Heart palpitates on exertion. Slept soundly.	No movement. Bowels painfully distended with flatus. Head mixed and confused. Swims on lying down. Heart palpitates on exertion. Feet and hands prickle. Less vigorous. Feels very weak. Ate well. Sleep disturbed with uneasiness in bowels. Legs and feet the same as on 25th inst.
28th.	Had no passage. Tongue clean, with red border and streak along centre. Appetite good. Considerable muscular debility. Numb feeling in head and extremities. Sleepy. Distended with flatus. Numbness and inability to control the feet and legs increasing.	No movement. Painfully disturbed with flatus, without ability to eructate or pass it. Head numb and mixed. Feet and hands prickle and are very numb. Heart palpitates on exertion. Flashes of chilliness and heat alternating. Losing control of lower extremities. Sleep disturbed.	At 11 a. m. had a scant constipated movement of pale, putty-like feces. Head numb and mixed. Feet and hands prickle. Heart palpitates on exertion. Tongue clean, red border. Full of wind during the night, which disturbed sleep. Feet and legs feel heavy and numb. Has less control over them than on 25th.
29th.	Throbbing heat about the rectum. Had a rather more free passage than usual during morning. Appetite good. Feels weak and debilitated. Considerable thirst. Bowels much disturbed with flatus during latter part of day, evening and night. Wakeful. Prickly numb feeling in feet, legs and hands. Walks with a shuffling gait; trips easily.	No movement. Bowels painfully disturbed with flatus, constantly in motion. Head bewildered and numb. Feels as if all the upper part were in a vise, and being squeezed. Feet and hands prickle. Heart palpitates on exertion and intermits. Oppressed breathing. Feels as if he could not get enough in his lungs to satisfy him. Often draws a long breath. Ate well. Sleep disturbed. Feet, legs and arms prickle. Feet and legs numb and losing control of.	No movement. Bowels painfully disturbed with flatus in constant motion. Head mixed and numb: feels as if a band were drawn tight around it. Feet and hands prickle. Heart palpitates. Weak and languid. Great thirst, which is quenched with cold water. Ate well. Wakeful. Extremities prickle and feel more or less numb, and heavy. Losing control of his legs and feet.
30th.	No passage. About the same symptoms as 29th. Wakeful.	Had a large passage of pale thin feces with much wind at 4 a. m. Felt greatly relieved. Ate well and slept soundly.	No movement. Bowels largely disturbed with flatus, producing much uneasiness. About the same symptoms as 29th. Ate well. Slept well.

DAY.	MR. H.	MR. B.	MR. S.
31st.	Quite a free passage during the morning. Considerable heat and throbbing in the lower bowels. Large quantities of flatus developed in stomach and bowels during the evening and night with eructations and passages of wind. Wakeful. Extremities have a numb feeling and gait unsteady. Losing use of legs.	Had a profuse, windy, yeasty movement at 6 a. m. which gave great relief. Heat and throbbing in the lower bowels. Bloated up much during the day and night. Head less numb and confused. Feet and hands still prickle. Ate well. Slept soundly. Gait unsteady. Legs and feet numb. Losing control of the lower extremities.	No movement. Bowels painfully disturbed with flatus. Head numb and mixed. Feet and hands prickle. Head swims on lying down. Quite bewildered at times. Heart palpitates on exertion. Flashes of heat alternated with chilly sensations. Feet and hands cold. Breathing oppressed. Ate well. Sleep disturbed. Gait unsteady. Feet and hands prickle and feel numb. Losing control of the lower extremities.
Nov. 1st.	Aroused about 4 a. m. with a severe bearing down pain in the lower bowels and a desire to go to stool. Had a copious passage which was thin and watery, and of a pale ash color. Passed large quantities of flatus. Heat and throbbing pain about the lower part of the large intestines. Small intestines and stomach disturbed with wind before the stool. The free passage relieved this, so that he fell asleep and slept till 7 a. m. Got up free from pain and feeling well save the weakness and disagreeable paralytic symptoms. Appetite good. Tongue clear, with red streak along the centre. Flashes of heat over the body, intermitted with chilly sensations. Bowels almost constantly disturbed with flatus. Much worse during evening and night. Retired early and slept well till 3 a. m. Gait unsteady. Mixed, confused feeling in the head. Extremities not fully under control.	Aroused at 3 a. m. with pain and commotion in lower bowels, followed by a profuse, bulky, windy, yeasty passage of pale, mushy feces. Would fill a chamber, but had but little weight. Heat and throbbing in lower bowels. Greatly relieved after the passage. Head less confused. Feels lighter and brighter. Fell asleep and slept till 7 a. m. Ate well. Bloated painfully during the day. Gait unsteady. Head mixed and confused, and memory bad. Extremities more or less numb and cold; he is losing control of them.	At 6 a. m. had a profuse, mushy, yeasty passage of a pale color, accompanied by much wind. Felt greatly relieved after. Ate well during the day. Bowels became painfully disturbed with flatus before night. Ate well. Slept soundly till 5 a. m. when he was aroused by a desire to have a passage. Had a profuse, bulky, mushy movement of pale color; would fill a chamber. With it came much wind, which greatly relieved the distention. Head less dizzy and numb. Feels brighter. Extremities prickle and feel numb. Losing control of legs and feet.
2d.	At 3 a. m. was awakened with a severe, bearing down pain in lower bowels, with an urgent desire to go to stool. Had a copious, watery discharge with much wind, which relieved the pains. Considerable heat and throbbing in lower bowels. Felt well during the day. Appetite good. Bowels disturbed with gas during the night. Gait unsteady. Losing use of the lower extremities.	Had a profuse passage of pale, bulky, mushy feces at 7 a. m., followed by a second of the same character at 8 a. m. With these passages much flatus was passed. Head mixed and confused. Unsteady in gait. Extremities prickle and feel cold and numb. He walks with difficulty.	Heat and throbbing pain in the lower bowels. Appetite good. Tongue clean with red streak along centre and around edges. Ate well and slept soundly. Extremities cold and feel numb. Gait unsteady. Head mixed and confused. Hard to collect his ideas and memory very poor.

DAY.	MR. H.	MR. B.	MR. S.
3d.	At 3 a. m. had another profuse passage of pale, foamy, watery feces. Considerable heat, bearing down and throbbing in rectum and descending colon. Much debilitated during the day, but appetite good and free from pain. Tongue clean, with a red streak along the centre that felt sore. On examining the feces with the microscope, found them full of yeast plants belonging to the genera Saccharomyces and Mycoderma, with all the products of fermentation developed by their growth, precisely as is found in the stools of consumption of the bowels, or Chronic Diarrhœa. During the afternoon, evening and night, the stomach and intestines were very much disturbed with gases, producing considerable pain. Wakeful. Gait unsteady. Extremities cold and numb. Cramps in legs.	Had a profuse, pale, bulky, mushy, yeasty passage at 3 a. m. accompanied by much wind. This was followed by another passage at 5 a. m. Another at 6 a. m. Another at 8.30 a. m. All were profuse, mushy and yeasty. On microscopic examination the passages were found filled with yeast plants belonging to the genera Saccharomyces and Mycoderma, with all the products of fermentation developed by their growth. After the passages there was much heat and throbbing in the lower bowels. The head, however, was much relieved of dizziness and numbness. During the afternoon and evening, the bowels became greatly disturbed with flatus. Ate well and slept soundly. Ideas quite confused. Extremities cold and numb. Gait very unsteady.	Had 4 profuse, yeasty, mushy passages between 4 a. m. and 10 a. m. All were light and very bulky, and filled with alcoholic and acid yeast plants, belonging to the genera Saccharomyces and Mycoderma. Felt greatly relieved after the movement. Head was less mixed. Confused and numb feelings. During the afternoon and night the bowels became greatly disturbed with flatus in constant motion. Ate well. Heart palpitates and intermits. Slept well. Head quite dizzy on rising. Gait unsteady. Extremities numb and cold. Drags the feet in walking.
4th.	Called up at 2 p. m. by a profuse passage of thin, pultaceous, pale, watery feces, with much wind. Between this and 10 a. m. had 6 profuse evacuations of the same yeasty, bulky, but light character: after this felt better. Fearing to carry the experiment further in this case I gave him, on retiring, a cathartic dose of Rochelle salts, which operated freely. Gait very unsteady. Not good use of lower extremities. Drags them in walking and has a wobbling walk. Marked symptoms of Locomotor Ataxy. Falls on closing the eyes.	Had a profuse, mushy, yeasty passage, accompanied by much flatus at 3 a. m. This was followed by 5 bulky, yeasty movements before 11 a. m. Was very much prostrated after these profuse evacuations, although felt much clearer and brighter. Gave a dose of Rochelle salts at 3 p. m. which operated freely. Slept well during the night. Cannot retain an upright position after closing the eyes. Head confused. Extremities cold and numb. Drags limbs in walking. Marked symptoms of Locomotor Ataxy.	Had a profuse, yeasty, mushy passage at 2.30 a. m. accompanied by much wind. Between this and 11 a. m. had 8 more profuse, yeasty movements which so prostrated him that he could hardly get out of bed. As the objects of this feeding had been accomplished, stopped the army biscuit diet and gave him a dose of Rochelle salts, which cleaned the yeast out of the bowels during the evening. Slept well. On rising found he could not stand upright on closing the eyes. Walks with a shuffling unsteady gait. Marked symptoms of Locomotor Ataxy.
5th.	Gave him a full breakfast of ham and eggs, with tea, and potatoes stewed in milk. Was ravenously hungry and ate a hearty meal, after which felt much better. Had no further evacuation after 10 a. m. during the 5th. At 3 p. m. ordered 6 soft boiled eggs, with water. These lay rather heavy on the stomach, producing some sour eructations. Ordered him to walk briskly for 2 hours, which made him feel much better. Retired at 9 p. m. feeling quite well. Slept soundly. Head clearing rapidly and gait becoming steady.	Gave him a full breakfast of ham and eggs, with tea, and potatoes stewed in milk. Was very hungry and ate ravenously, after which felt much better. Had 2 evacuations between 8 a. m. and 10 a. m. At 3 p. m. gave him a nice broiled steak, a cup of clear tea and a small piece of toast which he ate with great relish. Felt well. Took a brisk walk. Distention of bowels greatly lessened. Head less dizzy and numb. Feels brighter. Before night the bowels were again disturbed with flatus. Slept soundly.	Gave him for breakfast a nice broiled steak, a piece of toast and a cup of clear coffee. Ate a hearty meal with great relish. Felt well. Head quite clear and bowels but little disturbed with wind. At 3 p. m. gave him a large Porterhouse steak, a cup of clear tea and a slice of bread. Ate a hearty meal with great relish. Retired at 9 p. m. and slept well. Head becoming quite clear; gait much more steady. Numbness and coldness of extremities lessening rapidly.

DAY.	MR. H.	MR. B.	MR. S.
6th.	At 7 a. m. soon after rising, had a copious passage of thin, watery and rather pale feces, but looking much better than the passage yesterday morning. Under the microscope they had still the characteristic marks of chronic diarrhœa stools. There was considerable pain during the passage and previously, with heat and throbbing in the lower bowels afterwards, but no tenderness. Tongue clean, with red streaks along the centre and red edges. Made a hearty breakfast on ham and eggs, toast and tea, after which felt better. From this time on, he continued the albuminous, animal diet, eating freely. Appetite remarkably good, Each day improvement was noticed in the tone of the bowels, in the appearance of discharges, and in a lessened fermentative tendency in stomach and bowels. Decrease also in the alcoholic and acid yeasts, and gelatinous mucus from the large intestines, which is always present in Chronic Diarrhœa. Legs and feet warmer and less numb. Handles limbs better.	Had a profuse, yeasty, mushy passage, accompanied with considerable wind at 6.30 a. m. At 8 a. m. had a second passage; less bulky and yeasty and less wind with it. Ate 2 ounces of broiled steak for his breakfast, with small piece of toast, and drank a cup of clear tea. Head quite clear, and flatulence mostly gone. Feels quite well. For dinner gave him 1 lb. broiled steak, a slice of toast and a cup of clear tea. Somewhat bloated during afternoon, but no more movements. For supper had 12 ounces of steak, half a slice of toast and a cup of clear tea. Retired at 9 p. m. feeling well. Slept soundly. Lower extremities warmer. Numbness disappearing. Walks easier and more steadily.	Had 1 yeasty, mushy movement at 7.30 a. m. with considerable wind. No more movements during the day. Gave him 12 ounces of broiled steak for breakfast, 1 lb. for dinner and 12 ounces for supper, with half a slice of toast and a cup of clear tea at each meal. Somewhat flatulent towards evening, but otherwise feeling well. Head clear. Tongue clean and healthy in appearance, and prickling sensations gone. Retired at 9 p. m. Slept soundly. Numbness and coldness of lower extremities disappearing. Walks much more steadily.
9th.	By this date had quite recovered, so that the passages had assumed their normal appearance and consistency, and came on after this at their usual hour, to wit: every morning before breakfast. The tongue became natural in appearance; the countenance fresh, the biliary secretions healthy, and the feces lost all the characteristics of those of Chronic Diarrhœa.	Continued the same diet as given on the 6th up to the 9th. Ate heartily and greedily. All the time improving. Had only 1 movement on the 7th; 1 on the 8th and 1 on the 9th. The passage on the 7th was somewhat yeasty; that on the 8th less so, and the one on the 9th quite normal, it being quite free from yeast and the products of fermentation. Feels perfectly well.	Continued the same diet as on the 6th up to the 9th. Had only 1 movement daily. The one on the 7th was a little mushy and light, but the one on the 8th and that on the 9th were quite normal in appearance, and gave no evidences of yeast and the products of fermentation. Feels well.

Close of the Experiments.

On the evening of the 9th, after giving my boarders a good beefsteak supper, I paid them off and discharged them from a diet drill to which they had submitted with a good grace for 28 days.

These three subjects are all strong, healthy men in the prime of life, who had been used to the substantial diet of the active business men of our Western cities. From the commencement of the army-biscuit diet, up to the time when the discharges assumed a yeasty, chronic diarrhœa type, 19 days elapsed in one case, 18 days in the second and 20 days in the third case. The fermentative condition, and the production of alcoholic and acid yeast (Saccharomyces and Mycoderma), commenced and showed themselves in a marked degree on or about the 6th day, and increased until the army-biscuit diet was discontinued.

The first abnormal condition brought about by this diet was constipation, with a partial suppression of the biliary and intestinal secretions and lessened peristaltic action. This left the alimentary matters in the stomach and intestines an unusual time, during which fermentative changes were started. This fermentative condition increased daily, till the alimentary canal became filled with alcoholic and acid yeasts in a state of rapid multiplication and development, disengaging large quantities of carbonic acid gas which distended the bowels with flatus.

Just previous to the commencement of the diarrhœa and afterwards, there was a general paralytic tendency : this was especially marked in the intestinal walls, they losing their normal sensibility and contractility under the irritant and poisonous action of yeast plants, carbonic acid gas, vinegar and other products developed during the fermentation of the amylaceous alimentary matters. In severe forms of the disease produced by this kind of feeding, the large intestines and sphincter become frequently so paralyzed that the feces pass involuntarily. About the time the diarrhœtic discharges commenced, there came on a huskiness and hoarseness of the voice, and a dry, constricted feeling about the larynx and pharynx. This was accompanied by a scalded, smarting soreness of the throat, as if it were inflamed, which extended into the bronchial tubes, together with the secretion of a thick, ropy, sweetish expectoration and considerable night and morning cough, with oppression and tightness about the chest. On examining the throat and larynx, the surfaces were found to be whiter than usual, showing that the parts were more deadened than inflamed.

This affection differed from all colds, it being caused by partial death or paralysis, instead of by over-action or inflammation. It continued while the diarrhœa lasted. There was also palpitation of the heart and oppressed breathing, on any excitement. I have noticed the same pulmonary derangement in all well-marked cases of chronic diarrhœa, or consumption of the bowels.

During these experiments, the boarders were not allowed to perform any manual labor, or permitted to take any exercise besides the two to four mile walks, morning and evening. I was constantly with them, day and night, to observe all the symptoms and conditions; to make such tests and microscopical examinations as were necessary to determine the various states and changes that were taking place and to indicate the latitudes and departures from the normal state.

Had they been allowed to labor and take vigorous exercise, the fermentation and consequent consumption of the bowels would have been deferred to a later date. Vigorous exercise would have shaken and worked the food down out of the stomach into the small bowels, where it is digested, before any very serious fermentation had set in. Such as did set in, however, would have finally culminated in the disease as before, but under a much slower rate of progress.

On the tenth day of the feeding, all the men began to show quite evident signs of semi-paralysis of the nerves of the extremities. This gradually increased until the army-biscuit diet was discontinued. During the last few days of the feeding the symptoms of locomotor ataxy were strongly marked, and the disease was progressing with alarming rapidity. The eyes were growing more and more dim, and the deafness and ringing in the ears were becoming strongly manifested.

LII.

A FINAL WORD ON FOODS AND ON MEAT DYSPEPSIA.

THE foregoing descriptions of the results of continuous feeding upon one food at a time, with a view of determining what especial diseased states might be brought about by each food, in the human body, are sufficient to give a clear idea of the significance, scope and character of this painstaking work. To go through all my food experiments in detail would make this treatise far too voluminous to be read and studied, except as a work of reference. This would defeat my desire of getting it into the hands of as many students as possible in the opening of their career, directing their attention, as well as that of all earnest thinkers, whether in the profession or out of it, to the urgent necessity of dietetic reform, and to the real nature of most of our diseases, based as they are upon departure from dietetic laws indicated by the organic structure of man.

I will state in this connection, that bread, rice, wheaten grits, hominy, tapioca, sago, potatoes, green peas, string beans, green corn, beets, turnips, squash, asparagus and the various meats, have each been fed upon exclusively and continuously by from four to six men at a time, for from seven to forty-five days. The results in all cases were recorded and tabulated as in the preceding experiments.

Bread, rice, wheaten grits, hominy, sago, tapioca and potatoes have each been fed upon continuously for from forty to forty-five days, before serious diseases and symptoms were produced. These foods are very similar in their action upon the human body, and cause like derangements and pathological states. They sustain the organism far better, and can be borne longer, than any other vegetable aliment, before grave disturbances arise from their exclusive use. The diseased conditions and states finally induced by them are as follows : Flatulence, weak heart, oppressed breathing, singing in ears, dizzy head, headaches, lumbago, constipation first and afterwards chronic diarrhœa ; thickened large bowel, cold feet, numbness in extremities, and general lassitude and weakness. Were the exclusive feeding too long kept up, either consumption of the bowels, or lungs, or both may result; or either locomotor ataxy, Bright's disease, diabetes, paresis, or fatty diseases of liver, spleen, or heart might be the final outcome. Also goitre, ovarian tumors, uterine fibroids, fibrous growths and fibrous consumption may be caused by such feeding in course of time.

Green peas and string beans rank next to the seven foods above named in point of alimentary qualities. Green corn, turnips, beets and squash, cannot be subsisted upon for more than a very short period (when taken exclusively) before most unpleasant and more or less grave derangements ensue. Of all vegetables, asparagus is one of the most injurious when lived upon alone. Seven days is about as long as it would be safe to subsist upon this plant. The great efforts made by the kidneys to eliminate the asparagine, which overstimulates them, rapidly exhausts the vitality of the victim, and in a few days he is scarcely able to navigate.

The experiments upon meat feeding showed that meats, and especially beef and mutton, can be subsisted upon without resulting in diseased states, for a much longer time than can the best vegetable products under the same conditions. The reason of this is that the first organ of the digestive apparatus — the stomach — is a meat-digesting organ. I have had patients afflicted with grave diseases, thrive and become perfectly well upon beef. Many of them have continued this as an exclusive diet from three to four years, before bringing breads and vegetables into their diet list. Good, fresh beef and mutton stand at the head of all aliments as foods promotive of human health.

Eggs, fish, pork, veal, chickens, turkeys and game come in merely as side dishes: they may be subsisted upon singly for a limited time without bad results. All of these, however, if continued alone for too long a time, or if eaten in undue proportion constantly, may eventually produce meat dyspepsia, and various scorbutic conditions which are disagreeable and sometimes difficult to handle, and may result fatally. In meat dyspepsia there is more or less distress, oppression and load about the stomach, with usually a ball in the throat, and the "gulping of wind" that tastes like "rotten eggs" (Sulphuretted Hydrogen). With these symptoms there is frequently much sickness and weakness, with loss of appetite and great heat and bewilderment in the head. In treating this form of dyspepsia, all food by the mouth has to be discontinued, and nourishment given by the rectum till the stomach can be thoroughly washed out and disinfected. Then feeding by the mouth is carefully begun by giving a very small quantity of pulp of beef and bread foods at first, gradually increasing them as digestion improves.

LIII.

VINEGAR. ITS EXCESSIVE USE TENDS TO PRODUCE TUBERCULAR DISEASE.

IN cases where vinegar is drunk daily to reduce obesity, or for the satisfaction of a morbid appetite, the same kind of constipation, flatulence, diarrhœa, cough and disposition to tuberculosis and fibrinous depositions in the pulmonary capillaries and heart (as demonstrated by the foregoing experiments) will occur. Every observant physician has noticed the tendency which vinegar has — when taken largely and daily repeated — to produce irritation of the intestinal and pulmonary membranes, with diarrhœa and cough. Several cases of the kind are published in foreign journals. The following is one in point, taken from the London " Medical Gazette," Vol. 2, 1838–39 : —

" A few years since, a young lady in easy circumstances, enjoying good health, was very plump, had a good appetite, and a complexion blooming with roses and lilies. She began to look upon her plumpness with suspicion, her mother being very fat and she afraid of becoming like her. Accordingly she consulted a woman, who advised her to drink a small glass of vinegar daily; the counsel was followed and the plumpness soon diminished. She was delighted with the success of the remedy and continued it for more than a month. She began to have a cough, but it was at first dry and regarded as a cold that would subside. But from being dry, it was presently moist. A slow fever came on, with difficult breathing; her body became lame and wasted away; night sweats, with swelling of the feet, succeeded, and a diarrhœa terminated her life. On examination, all the lobes of the lungs were found filled with tubercles, and somewhat resembled a bunch of grapes."

LIV.

RESEMBLANCE BETWEEN THE COLLOID MATTER DEVELOPED IN CHRONIC DIARRHŒA AND THAT FORMED IN BRONCHOCELE AND OVARIAN TUMORS.

COLLOID disease arises from unhealthy alimentation, and there is a marked resemblance between the colloid matter developed in the stomach and intestines of chronic diarrhœa, and that formed in bronchocele and ovarian tumors.

In the valleys of Switzerland, where goitre is so common, the inhabitants live almost entirely upon vegetable food. This has been observed and particularly commented upon by travelers and others who are familiar with the people and customs of these Alpine valleys. The fact is interesting in this connection, since the colloid matter deposited in the *thyroid glands*, producing goitre, is closely analogous to or identical with colloid matter developed in the alimentary canal in chronic diarrhœa.

It has been determined by the preceding investigations that amylaceous food, its fermentation in the alimentary canal and the consequent development of sugar, carbonic acid, yeast plants and so forth (rendering the system highly glycogenic and fermentative), are the true causes of those abnormal systemic conditions in chronic diarrhœa which induce the development of colloid matter: it is also extremely probable that the colloid matter of bronchocele may have a similar cause or origin.

The fact that the inhabitants of the Swiss valleys, wherein goitre obtains, live mainly upon vegetable food, is strong evidence in support of this opinion. The same kind of colloid development occurs in the female breast and in the male testes, in certain diseased conditions of the system.

Bronchocele prevails in the Alpine valleys of Switzerland to a greater extent than at any other known point. It is also quite prevalent in certain parts of England, as in Derbyshire and Nottingham, from which fact the disease is known in these localities as "Derbyshire Neck." The disease occurs to a most remarkable extent in the deep, warm, damp, malarious valleys of the Rhine in Switzerland, and is also found in some similar valleys of France, Spain, Germany, Austria, England and South America. Wherever it is very common among the people, the hygrometric and other meteorological conditions are such as to particularly favor the development of low cryptogamic forms; fermentative changes are active, and the people are eminently vegetarians and often drink much sour wine. The disease is *colloid* in character.

Where a people are in the habit of a too exclusive use of amylaceous and vegetable food from infancy — especially in damp, low, malarious valleys — there seems to be a marked tendency to the development of goitre. There is also a disposition to colloid development in the testes and mammary glands, in the alimentary canal and the lining membrane of the urinary and genital organs, and to flatulence, sour eructations and indigestion. They are subject to diarrhœa, palpitations of the heart, to fibrinous depositions in the pulmonary capillaries, and to congestions in the lungs, brains and intestinal walls. They are also liable to impairment of voice, hearing and vision. Often the lower extremities give more or less indications of paralytic tendencies. Where the goitrous tendency is extreme, there is also present a liability for it to run into that extreme, idiotic, pitiable form of the disease denominated Cretinism. Goitre may make its appearance at any period of life, though more commonly the thyroid glands begin to enlarge in early years.[1]

Cretinism. — This never occurs except where goitre is very

---

[1] These investigations appear to throw valuable light upon a great variety of sarcomatous abnormal developments, and especially that type known as gelatinous sarcoma, and other colloid forms of disease. These appear to be expressions of certain systemic conditions which are abnormal, and must be corrected and the causes removed before such diseased developments can be checked.

prevalent. It is the extreme state of congenital colloid disease. It may not be confined to the thyroid glands, but frequently extends to the mammæ, testes, lining membrane of the alimentary canal, and that of the urinary and genital organs. It is congenital, the children being born idiotic and with thyroid tumors, more or less large, which often become immense as they advance in years. Such persons are anæmic and diminutive, the stature seldom being over four and a half feet and often less. The cranium is deformed and has a conical shape; the forehead thrown backwards, narrow and flat, and the occiput in a line with the neck. The lower jaw is long and prominent; its elongated form and the thick, padded lips of the Cretins making them resemble ruminating animals more than man. The tongue is thick, watery and hangs out of the mouth, which is open, large and slavering. The flesh is soft and flaccid; skin wrinkled, yellow, cadaverous, dirty and covered with chronic eruptions. The eyes are small but prominent, red, watery and frequently squinting; the pupils contracted and not very sensitive to light. The look is a fixed stare, without expression. The senses are more or less defective, or altogether abolished, the Cretin being often deaf and dumb. Those who possess the faculty of speech can only speak imperfectly and with difficulty. The hearing is always very defective. The external ear is large and stands out from the head. The abdomen is large, flatulent, prominent, *and is usually distended with gases* and largely developed towards the chest. The flesh of the extremities is flabby. The thyroid gland is always more or less enlarged, often enormously so. The other glands above named are also enlarged.

The Cretins are voracious and addicted to masturbation. They often pass the feces involuntarily. The genital organs are largely developed, the testes large, and the scrotum frequently extends to the knees. The mammæ are voluminous and pendent, the menses deranged and the powers of procreation defective. They seldom live beyond the age of thirty, and often die much younger. They are usually of lymphatic temperament, with light hair and gray eyes. Such persons have a peculiar affection for the sun, at which they gaze vacantly and steadily for hours together, as if it imparted to them an inexpressible pleasure. They may be said to be sun-worshipers by intuition.

The following interesting letter, relating to the diet and habits of people residing in the goitrous valleys of Switzerland, France and other countries, is from Professor Lesquereux, our justly famed fossil botanist. He is at home among the Alps, and is perfectly familiar with all the habits and customs of this interesting people. Therefore his statements are especially valuable in this relation, as when taken in connection with the observations and experiments heretofore given, they render it highly probable, if not certain, that the goitrous diathesis originated entirely from the vegetable diet of the people, aided by those meteorological conditions which favor the development of low cryptogamic forms : —

COLUMBUS, OHIO, *January 9*, 1864.

DR. J. H. SALISBURY.

MY DEAR SIR, — I am sorry that I am not able to answer all your inquiries concerning the symptoms generally accompanying the appearance and development of the goitre. I studied this peculiar sickness rather as a naturalist than a doctor would do it ; rather trying to analyze the peculiar causes of its appearance, than to analyze the various modifications to which different parts of the body are subjected. You want to know :

1. In what part of the country of Switzerland the goitre is mostly prevalent ?

2. What are the habits of the people mostly attacked by it ?

3. To what cause is the sickness generally attributed ?

1st. The goitre is mostly prevalent along the rivers and at the bottom of some deep valley of the Alpine mountains. I have observed it especially in the *Canton Vallais*, along the valley of the Rhone, from Sion to St. Maurice. I have seen it also on the Jura Mountains, near Montbeillard, in Franche-Comte, and also in some parts of Savoy, especially in the valley d'Aorta. The goitre does not attack the inhabitants of the mountains or of the high valleys of Switzerland. The valley of the Rhone presents a peculiar appearance. It is so deeply encased in high chains of mountains, that in winter the sun does not reach the bottom of some parts, near St. Maurice, for example ; and that in summer the reflection of the sun by the surrounding walls of rocks causes the heat to be excessive. In winter-time, and also in the fall, the valley is generally and constantly covered with a deep fog. Even in summer-time, as soon as the sun is down, the valley is covered with a deep fog.

The inhabitants of the Canton Valais, or Valesia, who live in high valleys, or on the slopes of the mountains somewhat above the Rhone, are not subject to the goitre, as I said above. These generally have a splendid development of the body, and the most healthy appearance.

It may be remarked, also, that along the valley of the Rhone, the goitre is mostly predominant among the inhabitants belonging to the Catholic faith. Thus, from St. Maurice downwards, the left side of the valley is Valaisian and Catholic — and there the goitre is very predominant. The right side belongs to the State of Vaud, and is Protestant. There are still some cases of goitre deformation, but no Cretinism whatever. This Cretinism appears to be the extreme point of development of the goitre. It is a kind of bodily deformity, accompanied with idiotism, presenting the most disgusting appearance. The Cretins are born idiots — generally from individuals either Cretins or affected with the goitre in its utmost development. They all bear a goitre of enormous size — sometimes descending on their stomach. They are of short size, no more than four feet high ; have a wrinkled, yellowish, pale, cadaverous skin, generally covered with a coat of filth ; some are blind, or deaf and dumb ; some have the itch or other ulcerous affections. Their eyes are red, protuberant and far between; their mouth is generally open, and outrunning with saliva; the visage flat and blue, the front very narrow and backward. They live in filth, are voracious, lazy and lascivious. They intermarry and generally live on the charity of the people.

2d. The inhabitants of the valley of the Rhone are poor. Their only industry consists in the cultivation of vineyards and of small farms. They are all of the Catholic faith, lazy and dirty. The poor ones mostly live on a kind of very black bread, made with the flour and bran of oats. They eat very little meat, if any, drink water and some of their acid wine, but no alcoholic liquors. Higher up in the mountains, and on their slopes, the inhabitants are richer, with their fine pastures and fine herds of cows. Their industry of cheese making is remunerative. These live especially upon milk in its various decompositions and preparations, and have no goitre. They are the most beautiful, kind and good people that it is possible to find. In the Swiss Jura Mountains, the poor of the inhabitants live mostly *on goat's milk ; and though they are not very clean, they have no trace of goitre, even in the deepest valleys.*

3d. The essential cause of the formation of *goitre* (of course I speak of causes appreciable to common observation) is the dampness of the atmosphere. This cause is not simple; it is confined with the filth in which the poor inhabitants of Valesia are generally living, and their poor and bad food. The sickness was at first attributed to water. But as the inhabitants of the mountains drink the same kind of water as those of the valleys, and have no *goitre,* it is obvious that the water has nothing to do with the development of the goitre. A damp atmosphere *can also not be considered as the sole cause of the sickness ;* for on the right side of the Rhone, below St. Maurice, the inhabitants, who are thrifty, rich and clean,[1] a Pro-

---

[1] Professor Lesquereux tells me that this Protestant people use more of a meat diet than the poorer class on the opposite side of the river, the food of which people is almost entirely vegetable.

testant population, have scarcely any goitre, and no Cretins whatever. *In Franche-Comte, near Montbeillard, on the contrary,
the locality where I have seen the goitre, is not a deep valley,
and there the dampness of the atmosphere cannot be considered as the essential cause. But here the inhabitants are
proverbially filthy, lazy and poor of course. The women cul-
tivate some patches of corn. Corn meal, prepared in a kind
of porridge, being their essential and sometimes their only
food.* This part belongs to France.

The Swiss Government has done much — not only to promote researches concerning the cause of the goitre and of Cretinism, but also to find the means of curing the poor idiots of
Valesia. A kind of hospital has been established under the
management of a celebrated doctor, in a high, open valley of
the Alps. There, good food, exercise, cleanliness and education
have done much, if not to extirpate this plague, at least to
alleviate and diminish its influence.

The inhabitants of Valesia, and of the countries where the
goitre is prevalent, do not appear to lose anything of their
strength by the mere development of the goitre. I have seen
most beautiful women and men, of the finest and most healthy
growth, attacked by it. Even in the valleys of the Pyrenees
and of the Alps, where the goitre is general, the inhabitants
who are not attacked by it are looked on' and pitied as a kind
of cripples, or of deformed beings, because they do not bear
under their chins this appendage probably considered as some
pleasant apparel.

I could write you much more on the subject; but I think
that this letter is long enough. Should you want an answer to
some other questions, I shall be always glad to tell you what I
know on the matter.

Very sincerely yours,   LEO LESQUEREUX.

LV.

EXPERIMENTS IN PRODUCING RHEUMATISM, THROMBOSIS, EM-
BOLISM, CONSUMPTION OF BOWELS AND LUNGS AND EN-
LARGEMENT OF LYMPHATIC GLANDS BY THE EXCESSIVE USE
OF VINEGAR.

IN November, 1863, I placed three strong, healthy men, myself making the fourth, on ordinary diet, with vinegar in sweetened water as an exclusive drink. The food consisted of boiled
and roasted meats, vegetables and bread for dinner and supper,
and hash, potatoes and bread for breakfast. The meats made
up about one twelfth the bulk of the vegetables and bread, which
is about the average proportion in which these foods are usually
taken. The only drink used was three ounces of strong cider
vinegar in half a pint of sweetened water at each meal to each
man, and the same amount from two to three hours after breakfast and dinner. This gave fifteen ounces of vinegar daily to
each person. These experiments began at noon on the tenth of
November, 1863. My results in feeding swine on the acid slop
of the whiskey distillery in 1858, had already prepared me to
be cautious to not carry these experiments too far, on account
of the danger of thrombosis, embolism, consumption and paralysis. The only exercise allowed was a walk of one hour, morning and evening. The men were constantly under my eye, and
every hour observations were made of the condition of each.
The two meals taken on the first day (Nov. 11th) produced no
unusual impression, save a slight watery and congested condition of all the mucous membranes.

First night all slept soundly and well. On the afternoon of
the second day, all began to feel more or less uncomfortable,

with flashes of heat and watery condition of eyes. Pulse accelerated : sour eructations with considerable flatulence, and constant movement of wind in the bowels.

In giving the results of these experiments in detail, I will designate the individuals of my household as A, B, C, and D.

DAY.	A.	B.	C.	D.
3	Considerable colic and very flatulent. Flashes of heat towards latter part of day. Bowels moved once. Urine flowed freely. Good appetite.	Some colic from constantly moving wind in bowels. Appetite good. Some fever, and watery condition of eyes. Face flushed.	Very flatulent and uncomfortable from moving wind in bowels. Face flushed. Watery secretion in eyes, nose and fauces. Constipated movement. Good appetite.	Very flatulent, with considerable colic at times. Flashes of heat, and watery condition of eyes and fauces. Appetite is good.
4	Bowels bloated, causing much discomfort, with increased heart's action on exertion. Appetite good. Eyes and fauces congested and watery. No movement. Sleep somewhat disturbed. Blood getting ropy and sticky. Urine free.	Much bloated and uncomfortable, with some oppression in breathing. Heart's action accelerated on exertion. Feverish at times. Mucous membrane of eyes, nose and fauces watery and congested. Tendency to sneeze. Urine free. Appetite fair. No movement.	Much bloated, very uncomfortable from colic and moving wind. Blood becoming ropy and sticky. Easily excited and nervous. Eyes and throat watery. Tendency to sneeze. Appetite good. Feels tired. No movement. Urine free.	Bowels bloated. Untus. Feels tired on exertion. Pulse accelerated, and easily excited. Blood becoming ropy and sticky. Eyes and nose watery. Appetite fair. Urine free. No movement.
5	Very flatulent with colic. Flashes of heat. Pulse 80 to 84. Easily excited. Rheumatic pains in knees and shoulders. Pain in region of heart. Eyes and fauces watery. Breathing oppressed. Constipated. Blood ropy, sticky, stringy. Vinegar yeast appearing in blood. Head mixed. Languid and feels tired on exertion. Stomach acid. Appetite only moderate. Sleep disturbed with dreams. Urine free but contains bile. Eyes and fauces congested and watery. Sneezing occasionally. Feverish. Perspiration sour.	Bowels much bloated. Colic pains. Sour eructations. Perspiration smells sour. Rheumatic pains in knees and ankles. Pulse 82 to 86. Flashes of heat. Breathing oppressed. Head mixed. Singing in ears. Appetite moderate. Blood very ropy, sticky and stringy. Vinegar yeast begins to show itself in blood. Small, hard movement of light-colored feces. Wakeful. Urine free and clear. Eyes and nose watery : appears as if he had taken cold. Some fever.	Bowels much distended with wind. Colic. Head mixed. Perspiration sour. Stomach sour. Breathing oppressed on exertion. Ringing in ears. Pains in knees, feet, shoulders and hands. Pulse 81 to 86. Appetite poor. Sleep disturbed with troubled dreams. Urine free, but rather high-colored. Blood very ropy, stringy and sticky. Small, dry, hard, light-colored passage. Eyes and fauces watery and congested. Flashes of heat.	Very flatulent and bowels much distended and colicky. Head confused. Acid eructations. Breathing oppressed on exertion. Ringing in ears. Pains in knees and fingers. Pulse 83 to 87. Urine high-colored, but quite free. Uneasy and restless through the night. Appetite fair. Blood very ropy and stringy. Vinegar yeast begins to show itself in the blood. Eyes and throat watery. Appears as if he had taken cold. Perspiration sour. Small, hard, light movement.

DAY.	A.	B.	C.	D.
6	Bowels distended with flatus. Colic pains. Sour eructations. Head mixed. Ears ring. Eyes and fauces congested and watery. Hacking cough at times. Blood very ropy, stringy and sticky. Pains in knees, feet, hands and shoulders. Shooting heart pains. Breathing oppressed. Perspiration sour. At times feverish. Urine high-colored, and moderate in quantity. Density 1.026. Breath sour. Vinegar yeast increasing in blood. Hard, small, light-colored movement, with much wind. Sleep disturbed. Pulse 85 to 88.	Bowels distended with flatus. Colic pains. Sour eructations. Head confused. Ears ring. Eyes, nose and fauces congested and watery. Hacking cough. Blood very ropy, stringy and sticky. Pains in knees, ankles, feet, hands and shoulders. Occasional heart pains. Pulse from 84 to 88. Breathing oppressed on exertion. Perspiration sour. Flashes of heat and chilly sensations intermit. Urine high-colored ; density 1.028. Breath sour. Vinegar yeast increasing in the blood. Small, hard, light-colored stool, followed by a looser one with much wind. Sleep uneasy. Neck glands begin to enlarge.	Bowels distended with flatus. Colic pains. Sour stomach. Head mixed. Ears ring. Eyes and fauces congested as with a cold, and watery, scalded sensation in throat. Blood stringy, ropy and sticky. Hacking cough. Pains in knees, ankles, feet, shoulders and hands. Shooting pains in heart. Pulse from 83 to 87. Breathing short and oppressed. Perspiration sour. Urine high-colored and scanty: density 1.029. Vinegar yeast increasing in blood. Small, hard, light-colored stool, followed by a loose one with much flatus. Very nervous. Sleep disturbed.	Bowels much distended with wind, giving colic pains. Sour eructations. Breath sour. Head mixed. Ears ring. Eyes and fauces congested, and watery. Face flushed ; feverish. Blood stringy, ropy and sticky. Hacking cough. Pains in all the joints of extremities. Shooting pains in heart. Pulse from 84 to 89. Breathing oppressed on exertion. Perspiration sour. Urine high-colored and scanty. Density 1.030. Vinegar yeast increasing in blood. Small, light, hard movement, followed by a loose one with wind. Sleep disturbed. Glands of neck begin to swell.
7	Bowels much distended with wind. Severe colic pains. Acid stomach; sour eructations. Head confused. Ringing in ears. Eyes, nose and throat congested and watery. Throat has a scalded, sore feeling. Coughs and expectorates a tough mucus. Blood very ropy, stringy and sticky. Pains in knees, feet, ankles, shoulders and wrists. Shooting heart pains. Oppressed breathing. Limbs prickle and get numb at times. Perspiration sour. Alternate fever and chills. Urine high-colored, scanty: density 1.030. Breath sour. Vinegar yeast increasing in blood. A small constipated passage, followed soon after by 2 loose movements. Sleep uneasy. Pulse 87 to 90. Neck glands swelling.	Bowels much distended with wind. Colic quite severe at times. Sour eructations. Singing in ears. Prickly feelings over bowels and in legs and arms. Eyes and fauces hot, watery and congested. Coughs frequently and expectorates a thick stringy and sticky, but less tenacious. Pains in all the joints of extremities. Breathing short and oppressed on exertion. Perspiration sour. Fever and chills alternately. Urine high-colored; density 1.031. Vinegar yeast increasing in blood. 2 loose movements of the bowels, in passing much wind. Pulse 88 to 92. Glands of neck enlarging.	Bowels distended with wind and full of pains. Acid stomach and sour eructations. Singing in ears. Prickly feeling in legs, arms and over bowels. Head mixed. Eyes and throat congested, hot, with a scalded feeling. Often has difficulty in swallowing. Cough quite severe. Expectorates a tough, ropy mucus. Blood ropy and sticky but less tenacious. Pains throughout the upper and lower extremities. Breathing at times labored and short. Diaphragm partially paralyzed. Heart aches. Urine high-colored: density 1.032. Vinegar yeast increasing in blood. 1 constipated movement, followed by 1 large, loose stool. Pulse 87 to 91. Glands of neck swelling.	Bowels very much distended with wind and painful. Sour eructations. Breath smells sour. Singing in ears increasing. Prickly feelings in upper and lower extremities and over bowels. A feeling of numbness in the head. Head confused. Eyes, nose and throat congested, with a scalded feeling in the latter. Hurts to swallow. Cough quite severe at times. Expectorates a tough mucus. Blood ropy, sticky and less tough. Pains over the entire extremities. Breathing short and at times labored. Breathes by elevating the shoulders, showing the diaphragm paralyzed. Pains in heart. Urine scanty and high-colored. Yeast increasing in blood. 2 loose, yeasty movements. Pulse 88 to 91. Neck glands swelling.

DAY.	A.	B.	C.	D.
8	Bowels very flatulent and full of pains. Stomach acid, with sour eructations. Head confused and aching. Ringing in ears. Staggers in walking. Eyes, nose and throat congested, as with a cold. Throat has a scalded feeling, with some difficulty in swallowing. Cough quite severe at times. Expectorates a tough, ropy mucus. Blood ropy and sticky, but less tenacious. Vinegar yeast increasing in blood. Pains in upper and lower extremities, with prickling and numbness. Head feels numb. Darting pains in heart. Oppressed breathing on exertion. Perspiration sour. Alternate fever and chills. Urine high-colored and scanty. Density 1.032. 2 profuse, loose, yeasty movements. Sleep disturbed. Pulse 88 to 92. Glands of neck considerably swollen and tender. Trip-hammer pulsations beginning to show themselves, indicating fibrous deposits in and near the heart.	Bowels very much distended and painful. Sour eructations. Head dizzy and confused; shooting pains through it. Ringing in ears. Reels in walking. Eyes, nose and throat congested, as with a cold. Throat has a scalded feeling, making it painful to swallow at times. Cough quite troublesome, expectorating a tough mucus. Blood ropy, sticky, but less tough. Vinegar yeast increasing in blood. Severe rheumatic pains in legs and arms, with numbness and prickly sensations. Heart pains. Breathing short and labored on exertion. Perspiration sour. Alternate fever and chills. Urine high-colored and scanty; density 1.031. 3 loose, yeasty movements. Pulse 89 to 93. Slept uneasily. Glands of neck tender and much swollen. Heart beating spasmodically at times with trip-hammer tendencies, indicating the beginning of Thrombosis.	Bowels very much distended and achy; a cold, prickly feeling over them. Head dizzy and mixed. Ringing in ears. Unsteady on legs. Eyes, nose and throat hot, congested and watery, as with a cold. Hurts to swallow. Coughs quite severely at times. Expectorates a tough mucus. Blood ropy and sticky, but getting less tenacious. Vinegar yeast increasing in blood. Severe rheumatic aches in all the joints, with shooting neuralgic pains in long bones; legs, arms, bowels and head prickly and feel numb. Breathing short and hurried on exertion. Perspiration sour. Alternate chills and fever. Urine high-colored and scanty; density 1.032. 3 yeasty, loose movements. Pulse 90 to 92. Submaxillary and neck glands tender and swollen. Heart beating spasmodically with marked intermissions.	Bowels very much distended, and full of pains; constant rumbling of gases. Prickly feeling over bowels and in head and extremities. Ringing in ears. Quite dizzy and confused. Throat has a scalded, sore feeling that makes it difficult to swallow at times. Coughs a tough, ropy mucus. Blood very ropy, and sticky, but less tough. Vinegar yeast increasing in the blood. Severe rheumatic pains in all the joints, with numbness. Breathing oppressed and short on exertion. Alternate chills and fever. Urine high-colored and scanty: density 1.031. 3 loose, large, thin movements. Pulse 89 to 92. Salivary and neck glands much swollen and tender. Trip-hammer pulsations marked, fibrinous depositions, or the beginning of the formation of thrombi.

On the morning of the ninth day, all were in such a forlorn, used up, miserable condition, that it was deemed advisable to bring these experiments to an end, for fear of some serious result. All had a profuse diarrhœa, having two or three large, yeasty movements each, before time for rising. In all the cases the heart-beat was becoming more or less intermittent and spasmodic, with trip-hammer pulsations, and the numb and dizzy feelings were increasing. I accordingly ordered a breakfast of broiled beefsteak. An hour before the meal, each one drank a goblet of hot water, in which was dissolved two drams of bicarbonate of soda. This sweetened the stomach and made all feel more comfortable. The breakfast was relished, each having a broiled beefsteak and a cup of clear tea. Between 6 a. m. and 12 m., each had from three to four large, profuse and yeasty movements, which cleaned out the bowels so that all were greatly relieved from flatulence, oppressed breathing and colic pains.

One and a half hours before dinner, each drank two goblets of hot water, in which were dissolved three drams of bicarbonate of soda, with great relief. Ordered for dinner broiled beefsteak and a cup of clear tea, which all enjoyed. The afternoon was one of comparative comfort, as we were all quite free from flatulence, rheumatic pains, numbness and oppressed breathing. One and a half hours before supper, each drank two goblets of hot water in which were dissolved three drams of bicarbonate of soda, which made the stomachs quite sweet and comfortable. Ordered for supper broiled steak and a cup of clear tea for each, which all enjoyed very much. Half an hour before retiring, each drank two goblets of hot water, in which were dissolved two drams of bicarbonate of soda. Retired at 9 p. m. in an enjoyable frame of mind. Had a restful night. On the morning of the tenth day, all were called at 5 a. m. to take two goblets each of hot water in which three drams of bicarbonate of soda were dissolved. This was taken in bed, after which we all rested for an hour, and then had a breakfast of beefsteak and clear tea, which was greatly relished. No movements of the bowels till after breakfast, when each had from two to three profuse, but much less yeasty movements between this time and 11 a. m.

All were feeling remarkably well and almost free from the confused, numb and painful feelings. The troublesome flatulence had disappeared. One and a half hours before dinner, each drank two goblets of hot water in which were dissolved three drams of bicarbonate of soda. Had for dinner beefsteak and clear tea, which were greatly enjoyed. No more movements of the bowels. One and a half hours before supper, each drank two goblets of hot water in which were dissolved three drams of bicarbonate of soda. Supper at 6 p. m., of beefsteak and clear tea. All ate heartily and felt exceedingly well. Half an hour before retiring, each drank two goblets of hot water in which were dissolved two drams of bicarbonate of soda. Retired with comfortable stomachs and clear heads. Had a refreshing night's sleep.

Awakened at 5 a. m. on the eleventh day to drink the hot water and bicarbonate of soda. At 6 a. m. had a breakfast of beefsteak and clear tea, which was greatly praised and much relished. After breakfast all were feeling so well, having had no movements of the bowels, flatulence, aches or dizziness, that it. was thought best to close the experiments. After paying off my boarders, I must say we parted with no small degree of reluctance, having suffered and almost died together, after which we recuperated on a few reparative and much relished meals of broiled steak.

LVI.

Date and Locality of Investigations.

In 1858 I began the study of Alimentation, or the effects of different kinds of food — where too exclusively or persistently used — upon the animal body.   My first labors in this direction were connected with the disease known as " Hog Cholera," and were carried on mainly at Newark, Ohio, at the distillery of Henry Smith, and at the pens of Smith and Wing.

They were constantly feeding at this time about 1,200 hogs. In addition to the examinations at this place, I visited the pens of Mr. Gibson, and those of Mr. Gough, the former at Richmond and the other at Aurora, both near Cincinnati, Ohio.

The same disease, under the same conditions, prevailed at both these localities, — only to a greater extent, — and the postmortem and microscopic indications were identical with those made at Newark, Ohio.   I also visited several localities where hogs were dying with the same disease, and where they were turned loose in cornfields and found feeding largely on the moulding, sour and fermenting tramped-down corn.   In no instance was I able to find hogs dying with the disease when they were being fed on good, sweet, unfermenting and unfermented food.

The Extent to which the Disease prevailed.

The disease had been for many years growing more and more fatal, and becoming more and more widely spread, — as slop (the slop from whiskey distilleries) feeding increased, — till at the time of the commencement of these labors, the percentage of deaths among hogs fattened on whiskey slop ranged from 20 to 80 per cent. The average would not fall below 25 per cent. The number of still-fed hogs — throughout the country — fattened annually, was about 7,500,000. 25 per cent. of these, or 1,875,000, died yearly. The average weight of each would be about 170 lbs. This would be 318,750,000 lbs., which would be equal to about $11,156,250. I mention these facts to show how important a matter it was to find out the cause and remedy for the disease. It was this that led me to undertake the investigation. I worked with the disease for many months, devoting my entire time to it, and made over 100 careful postmortem examinations, where microscopic observations and chemical tests were resorted to, to aid in arriving at more correct and satisfactory results. In studying the contents and condition of the stomach and bowels, the blood, the glands, the lungs and all the other parts where there were any abnormal indications, the microscope was a most valuable assistant. This disease is not confined to " slop-fed " hogs, but extends as well to those fed on sour, fermenting and mouldy corn. It is the custom in many portions of the Western States to allow the hogs to harvest the corn crop, — that is, when the corn crop becomes ripe enough to feed ; — instead of gathering, husking and feeding it, the hogs are turned into the field of corn and allowed to help themselves. Usually a temporary fence is run through the field, — cutting off a portion of it, — and into this part the hogs are turned. When all the corn is eaten, the fence is moved, so as to give the hogs access to more, and so on. The result of this kind of feeding is, that the hogs usually tramp down more corn than they eat.

This trampled corn becomes mixed with the soil ; rains dampen it ; the corn begins to ferment, mould and become sour, and the hogs are in great part compelled to feed on fermenting, sour and mouldy corn. It is not long after commencing to feed on this kind of food, before they begin to get more and more constipated and to bloat up with carbonic acid gas. After 2 or 3 weeks, chronic diarrhœa or consumption of the bowels (Hog Cholera) sets in, and from the third to the eighth week many hogs are lost with the disease known as " Hog Cholera."

The immediate cause of death, however, is usually thrombosis and embolism, as will be seen by the results given farther on. The cause of disease is the fermenting, sour food eaten.

Natural History of the Disease and Period of Susceptibility.

When the hogs are first put on either the fermenting and sour slop or corn, they eat ravenously for a few days. After a day or two they become very much constipated and bloated up with the carbonic acid gas developed from the fermenting food in the stomach and bowels. This constipation continues for from one to three weeks, when yeast diarrhœa or consumption of the bowels sets in, in all the hogs, and they have from ten to forty — and sometimes more — thin, yeasty, windy movements in twenty-four hours. The ravenous appetite, which they had at first, soon passes away, and they eat more daintily and begin to fall off in weight. This falling off in weight continues till after the eighth week, when those that are still alive begin to feed better and fatten rapidly. After the diarrhœa sets in, they soon begin to die, and the deaths continue to the end of the eighth week.

The greatest percentage of deaths occurs from the beginning of the fourth to the beginning of the seventh week. Paralytic symptoms begin to show themselves very soon after the bloating and constipation set in, and gradually increase — usually — till past the eighth week, when as those that survive begin to thrive, these symptoms grow less and less marked. The paralytic tendency is indicated by a gradual weakening in the limbs, labored breathing on exercising even moderately ; in a tendency to stagger and reel, and often in a dragging in the hind legs, and ringing in the ears. This latter state is made manifest by frequent shaking of the head, and if it be more on one side than the other, the side most affected is held the lowest, the ear lopping. These symptoms all become greatly aggravated in the later stages of fatal cases, the animals losing control over all the posterior portions of the body so that they are often unable to walk or even stand without support.

Cause and Pathology.

The immediate causes of death are *Thrombosis and Embolism.* These are produced by the large amount of acetic acid, either already in the slop, or developed in it in the digestive apparatus after being eaten.

This being taken up in large quantities, produces first a plastic, sticky condition of the blood, with a shortening in the fibrin filaments, which lessens the size of the meshes in this material in the blood-vessels; or in other words it produces a plastic and partially clotted state of the blood, and renders shreds of fibrin, and sticky colorless corpuscles, liable to adhere to the sticky walls of blood-vessels, thus forming a nucleus for a thrombus. The thrombi usually form in the region of the heart, and when they get sufficiently large and long to extend either into or through the cavities of the heart, — thereby preventing the valves from properly closing, — " trip-hammer " or violent spasmodic pulsations of this organ set in, to dislodge the thrombi. When these set in, nothing can save the life of the hog, death being only a matter of a few hours, or, at most, a few days.

As soon as the thrombi are loosened (or any portion of them), they rush along in the blood stream as emboli, till they reach the capillaries — or small blood-vessels — in some organ or organs, where they lodge, damming up the blood stream, and producing congestion, extravasation and often the rupture of blood-vessels, and inflammation. Death of course soon results. The organ in which these emboli lodge is determined by the location of the thrombi. In the majority of cases, this organ will be the lungs. The next most frequent place is the intestinal walls. Occasionally the muscles, brain, kidneys, etc., are the seat of embolism. This thrombosis and embolism — although the immediate cause of death — constitutes only a fatal sequence in the disease. The disease proper is produced by fermentation, and the passage of the products of this fermentation into the blood and tissues. After the trip-hammer pulsations begin, the body becomes more or less paralyzed; especially is this the case with the hind legs and all the posterior part of the body, which becomes unsteady and reels from side to side in walking. In fact, this partial paralysis begins to show itself very early in the disease, before the diarrhœa sets in. There is evidence of ringing in the ears, from the fact that the animal carries his head tipped to one side and every few minutes shakes his head. The eyes become affected, so that there is always (in the later stage of the disease) more or less blindness. The appetite is fair, but not ravenous, till the trip-hammer pulsations begin, when they cease to eat. They have more or less cough after the third week; their limbs and muscular system become feeble, and any — even moderate — exercise by driving or otherwise, is apt to produce pulmonary congestions and trip-hammer pulsations of the heart, which are followed by early death.

All still-fed hogs have this disease — " consumption of the bowels." Only those die, however, which do not eliminate the acid product of fermentation sufficiently fast to prevent its clotting the blood and resulting in the formation of thrombi in the blood-vessels. All those that survive the eighth week are eventually able to eliminate the acid produced, fast enough to prevent it from accumulating in the blood apparatus sufficiently to clot the blood and form thrombi. These survivors begin to eat well and fatten rapidly, though the bowels remain more or less loose. Notwithstanding this rapid fattening, the lymphatic glands enlarge more or less in all the hogs, and few or many tubercles are deposited and found in the lungs and intestinal walls, while any severe exercise by driving or running, often results in congestions in lungs or bowels. The more acid the slop, the greater the percentage of deaths caused by thrombosis and embolism. Those that survive the eighth week, though they now begin to thrive, and take on fat rapidly, are yet systemically enfeebled and present many evident signs of a diseased condition. The skin becomes red and erythematous over the whole body; the hair falls off either partially or almost entirely; scrofulous sores and tubercular swellings appear; they have more or less cough, with paralytic tendencies in their posterior parts. If it were not for the fact that the hogs are slaughtered after a few months' feeding, they all (if kept on this kind of food), or a large percentage of them, would die of consumption. *Hog Cholera is chronic diarrhœa or consumption of the bowels.*

The same causes that produce this disease, when continued long enough to permit the vinegar yeast (mycoderma aceti) to get into the blood apparatus and multiply there, sooner or later result in tubercular phthisis. The continuous and persistent supply of fermenting materials to the digestive apparatus, — after it has become a " first class," well-established " yeast pot," — keeps up a constant supply of the products of fermentation in the alimentary canal. The carbonic acid gas little by little paralyzes the cells of the follicles and villi, so that their normal selective power is soon impaired. It is by virtue of this power that the tissues receive their requisite nourishment (all unnecessary matters being rejected and passed off as excrementitious), and in its suspension the follicles and cells of the villi gradually begin to take up yeast, carbonic acid gas, acetic acid and other deleterious materials. After a time the whole system is thus saturated with fermenting elements and their products. In this abnormal systemic condition, spores of the genus Saccharomyces are often found developing in the cuticle and follicles of the skin: spores of the Mycoderma are also found in all the mucous membranes and in the blood apparatus. So soon as the products of fermentation begin to be taken up, the system slowly yields to the invasion of a partial paralysis. This is indicated by gradual weakening of the heart's action ; by loss of muscular power in the diaphragm, so that breathing is performed more and more by the elevation of the shoulders ; by the increased feebleness and acceleration of the pulse ; in short, by the exhaustion and enervation of the entire organism. This affects the heart and organs of respiration until they too are enfeebled, paralyzed and imperfectly nourished, while the tissues lose their normal strength, and soften so that the blood-vessels are liable to rupture, when bleeding ensues. These states are aggravated by the acid developed in fermentation, which partially clots the blood in the vessels, making it ropy and sticky under the action of the weakened heart ; this condition of the blood renders the subject liable to congestions. In this disease, the fibrin filaments become weakened, so that the clots formed in consumptive (phthisis) blood are soft and "rotten," [1] so to speak, while in rheumatism the fibrin filaments are strong and the clots firm and tough.

Post-Mortem and Microscopic Examinations.

The following statements are copied from my note-book and are the records made at the time of the examinations : —

---

[1] In Hog Cholera — or consumption of the bowels in hogs, and in chronic diarrhœa — or consumption of the bowels in man, — where they are quickly produced by too exclusive feeding on sour and fermenting food, and where the disease sets in in the bowels before seriously invading the blood glands and lung tissues, — the blood clots are tough and the fibrin filaments are comparatively strong. As soon, however, as the yeast spores (alcoholic and vinegar yeast) invade the blood glands (mesenteric and lymphatic glands and spleen), the blood-vessels and lung tissue, the colorless corpuscles formed in the blood glands begin to get sticky, plastic, spongy, swollen and soft, so that the fibrin filaments formed from them are also swollen, soft and rotten, and the resultant clots are wanting in normal toughness and easily broken down. This is the reason why there is so much weakness in the fibrous tissues in consumptive diseases and also why blood-vessels are so prone to rupture in the lung tissue. In such cases the food indicated for man is pure lean meat, pure fibrinous food, and the avoidance of all alimentary material that will ferment with alcoholic and vinegar yeast. In this way the yeast is checked in its development and is gradually eliminated : the weakened, almost destroyed fibrinous tissue receives its proper nourishment, becomes stronger, and by degrees returns to its normal condition.

Oct. 4, 1858. Six hundred and twenty-four hogs, purchased of the farmers in the surrounding country, were placed in the pens. All were healthy and in good condition. Their weight ranged from 100 lbs. to 300 lbs. each. Average weight about 170 lbs. They were immediately placed upon the slop from the distillery. All ate ravenously and seemed to be very fond of the new diet.

Oct. 5. Hogs begin to bloat and become more constipated; still eating ravenously.

Oct. 6, 7, 8. Bloating and constipation constantly increasing: still eating up clean all that is given them. Passages becoming dark-colored, very hard, scanty and infrequent.

Oct. 9, 10, 11, 12. Bloating and constipation increasing daily. Appetite falling off little by little. Passages scanty, seldom, hard and dark, accompanied with much wind. So bloated that they appear to be uncomfortable and uneasy. Appetite fair, but growing less and less ravenous.

Oct. 13 to 19. Constipation and bloating increase gradually; dizziness, ringing in the ears and slight reeling in the posterior parts begin to show themselves, indicating paralytic tendencies. Appetites much less ravenous, but fair.

Oct. 20. Constipation giving way to diarrhœa. All the hogs begin to manifest signs of looseness, and a few are down with severe yeast diarrhœa. Passages in those that have diarrhœa, of a light color, windy, yeasty, thin, bulky and profuse. Appetites less ravenous. One hog was noticed this morning with the " trip-hammer " pulsation in side. It refused to eat, was partially paralyzed, reeling in walking, with the nose to the floor, head held to one side and shaking it frequently. Indifferent to its surroundings, and appears to be partially deaf and blind. At 10 a. m. it fell over on its side; surface became blue, breathing short and labored, and heart beating spasmodically. Died at 12 m.

Oct. 21. Diarrhœa increasing in all the hogs. Appetites lessening, and a marked falling off in condition; bloating going away and passages frequent, yeasty, thin and profuse. Three hogs died to-day with thrombosis and embolism.

Oct. 22. Diarrhœa increasing, appetites lessening and hogs falling off in weight. Begin to look lank and sickly. Four hogs died to-day after suffering with the " trip-hammer " pulsation of heart for from 6 to 12 hours. All become cyanotic and very much oppressed for breath and paralyzed before death.

From Oct. 23 to Nov. 2, 38 hogs died of " Hog Cholera," all of which survived from 6 to 18 hours after the " trip-hammer " pulsations set in. During this time the diarrhœa was constantly increasing and the hogs were constantly falling off in weight.

Nov. 2. Three hogs died last night and to-day. Commenced making post-mortem examinations.

CASE I. Weight about 140 lbs. Suffered with "trip-hammer" pulsations of heart for 12 hours before death. Surface blue. As soon as dead, opened the body. Heart was still spasmodically contracting and jerking, although entirely emptied of blood. Pericardium and heart seemed healthy and natural, aside from a thrombus extending into and partially through the organ.

Lungs. The upper lobes and posterior portions were congested, softened and blackened with extravasated blood. The anterior and lower portions were also congested, but so recently and partially that no extravasation had taken place. Cavity of chest contained about three ounces of effused bloody serum.

Diaphragm. Congested and inflamed.

Stomach. Vessels of, congested and enlarged. Cavity empty, and covered with slimy, offensive mucus. A microscopic examination of the contents of the stomach and intestinal canal determined the presence of the minute spores of the acetic ferment. (Mycoderma Aceti.)

Symptoms before Death. Was taken with " trip-hammer " pulsations of heart 12 hours before death. As soon as these began, he ceased to take food, became listless, dumpish and insensible to surrounding objects; held his nose down to the floor, eyes dull, heavy and glossy; staggered about, hardly able to support itself upon its legs. Soon the surface became blue, the hind portion of the body paralyzed, and the animal, unable longer to walk, fell over on its side and soon expired.

CASE II. Nov. 3. Cool and wet in morning. Temperature throughout the day from 40° to 45° Fah. 3 hogs died last night, that were noticed sick for first time yesterday. The 3 following are the ones.

Has been dead several hours, body cold. Died sometime during last night. Post-mortem 10 a. m.

Lungs. Completely congested, — with air cells filled with exuded, clotted blood, and frothy serum and mucus. Blood and mucus extend up into windpipe, (which was readily pulled out,) in a clot, 8 inches long, exhibiting a perfect cast of the trachea.

Heart. Quite natural, except in having two long ropes of attached fibrin (thrombi) extending through the organ. Kidneys and brain not examined. Diaphragm congested and inflamed. Stomach highly congested and very much inflamed and softened. Contained ropy mucus and small quantity of fermenting food. Microscopic examinations revealed minute tubercular deposits in walls of small intestines and in the upper portions of both lungs. The blood was filled with masses of the spores of the mycoderma aceti, and the fibrin was in a clotted condition throughout the blood apparatus. This hog died of embolism of the lungs.

CASE III. 12 m. Nov. 3. Body cold. Lungs less congested and inflamed than in the previous case, but sufficiently so to cause death. Vessels of lungs were filled with clots, — emboli, — the heart contained a large thrombus and the stomach was highly congested with clotted blood. The other organs were healthy, except the large bowels, which were thickened and filled with ropy mucus and fermenting food. The microscopic examinations revealed the same condition of blood, lungs and bowels as in Case II.

Case IV. Body cold. The left lung has been so long congested and inflamed, that it was entirely useless, filled with exuded, clotted blood and mucus, and softened. The right lung was highly congested and inflamed in the upper and back portions. The front and lower portion were more slightly and more recently affected. Stomach congested and inflamed; vessels enlarged and filled with clotted blood. Intestines inflated with gases, slightly congested and containing considerable ropy mucus and some fermenting food. Other organs healthy. Surface of body blue. The microscopic examination revealed minute tubercular deposits in lungs and walls of bowels. The contents of bowels and stomach were filled with the spores of the mycoderma aceti, as was also the blood. This hog, like the three preceding, died of thrombosis and embolism, caused by the acid of the fermenting slop.

Case V. Died at 11 a. m., Nov. 3. Was noticed sick late last evening. Became partially paralyzed at 8 a. m. this morning. Spasmodic beating of heart, not as severe as the preceding cases. Post-mortem at 3 p. m. Body cold. Surface not blue; quite natural. Blood seemed to be arterialized up to time of death.

Brain. Meningeal vessels and sinuses of brain gorged with blood.

Pericardium. Filled with bloody serum. Contained about one quart of exuded matter. Heart was black and covered with exuded clotted blood, and contained several small thrombi. Fibrin partially organized and deposited on the surface of heart and walls of pericardium. Every indication of a high state of inflammation of heart. Substance of heart hardened and enlarged.

Lungs. Right lung highly congested, inflamed and swollen.

Color dark; texture soft; appears to have been congested for many hours before death. Left lung quite healthy, or sufficiently so to arterialize the blood up to the moment of death.

Diaphragm. Engorged with blood and inflamed. Serous lining of chest on left side highly congested and inflamed. Stomach inflated with gases, congested, inflamed and filled with ropy mucus and yellow watery matter. Liver quite healthy. Kidneys internally filled with clotted blood; outside, light colored. Mesentery and intestines congested. Death in this case arose from thrombi in heart, and emboli in left lung. The microscopic examinations revealed embolism of left lung and vessels of pericardium. Blood filled with small masses of the spores of mycoderma aceti, and the contents of bowels filled with the spores of Mycoderma and Saccharomyces. The mesenteric glands were enlarged, and the walls of bowels contained minute tubercular deposits.

CASE VI. Died at 12 m., Nov. 3. Was noticed sick for the first time on the evening of the 2d. Surface slightly blue before and after death. Staggered as it walked, for several hours before death, — exhibiting the characteristic reel of the posterior part of the body. Post-mortem 4 hours after death. Body cold. Pericardium contained about 3 ounces of bloody serum. Heart contained a thrombus. Lungs, both congested and inflamed, and air cells filled with exuded clotted blood and mucus. Stomach highly congested around the pyloric extremity. Other portions quite healthy in appearance. Filled with mucus and a yellowish, watery, fetid matter. Kidneys slightly congested, and contained small clots of blood. Liver, spleen and small intestines slightly congested. Meningeal vessels and sinuses gorged with blood. *Microscopic examinations:* Found embolism of lungs, pericardium and meningeal vessels. The upper lobes of both lungs contained many tubercles. The blood contained spores of the mycoderma aceti, and the contents of stomach and bowels were filled with yeast vegetation like that in the slop.

CASE VII. Nov. 4. Sunday, 8 a. m. Cold and windy. Temperature from 32° to 35° Fah. "Trip-hammer" pulsations of heart first noticed yesterday morning. Died last night. Still warm. Surface not blue. Brain congested. Meningeal vessels and sinuses gorged with blood. Intestines highly congested and inflamed in their whole length, and blackened. Mesentery congested, inflamed and covered with clots of exuded blood. All the large vessels (internal) gorged with clotted blood. Kidneys inflamed and pelvis filled with clotted blood. Left lung congested and filled with clotted blood, blackened. Right lung only partially congested, not sufficiently so as to prevent the arterialization of the blood up to the moment of death; hence the surface of the body did not present the usual blue appearance. Pericardium contained about two ounces of bloody serum. Thrombus in heart. Liver somewhat congested. Cavity of chest and abdomen contained about one quart of exuded bloody serum and froth. Stomach somewhat congested, inflamed and filled with fermenting food and a dark green, slimy mucus. The animal died of embolism of meninges, mesentery, intestines and pericardium. This hog had been suffering with chronic diarrhœa, or consumption of the bowels, for about three weeks before the thrombosis was made manifest by "trip-hammer" pulsations of heart. As these clots were dislodged by the violent beating of the heart, they were carried along in the blood stream till lodged in capillaries and small blood-vessels of mesentery, intestines, pericardium and meninges of brain. All the preceding cases have been suffering like the last, with chronic diarrhœa for about three weeks previous to death.

CASE VIII. Died 8 a. m., Nov. 4, having been laboring under a severe diarrhœa for about three weeks, and with "trip-hammer" pulsations of heart for the last fourteen hours before death. Was very sluggish yesterday afternoon, with the nose to the floor, and reeling from side to side in walking. Refused to eat, appeared to be blind and deaf. Surface of body blue.

Post-mortem 10 a. m. Body still warm. Weight 200 lbs., and in good condition. Surface blue. Brain highly congested. Meningeal vessels gorged with clotted blood. Pericardium filled with serum. Serous membrane covering the heart covered with a mammillary deposit of partially organized fibrin. Color of a whitish blue. No exuded blood. Heart contained a thrombus. Left lung completely filled with clotted blood and mucus ; swollen, blackened and softened, with an odor of decay. Right lung considerably congested so as to be rendered quite useless before death. Upper portions of lungs filled with tubercles. Vessels of intestines filled with clotted blood, almost to the extent of bursting. Stomach highly congested and black with clotted blood. Filled with fermenting food and mucus. Kidneys blackened and filled with small clots of blood. Liver congested and blackened. Diaphragm congested and apparently gangrenous in spots. Death caused by thrombosis and embolism.

The Microscopic Examination.

Cut off the ears ten hours before death, and soon after the "trip-hammer" pulsations began. The surface was already blue. The blood was so thick it would not flow, but barely oozed out and piled up in a thick dark clot, which showed plainly that it was already clotted in the vessels. It was found full of small masses of the spores of mycoderma aceti. The same vegetation, with many spores of Saccharomyces, filled the fermenting contents of bowels.

CASE IX. Nov. 4. Was taken with "trip-hammer" pulsations in heart, yesterday. Had been suffering with chronic diarrhœa for twenty days previous. Died this morning. Weight, 200 lbs. — 12 m. Body still warm. Surface blue. Meningeal vessels gorged with black, clotted blood. Pericardium with one quart of bloody serum. Surface of pericardium, inside, covered with granules and strings of partially organized fibrin. Color of heart, black and bloody outside. Thrombus inside. Left lung black and perfectly covered and filled with clotted blood; softened and enlarged. Air cells filled with clotted blood and froth. Right lung highly congested and filled with clotted blood, but more recently involved than the left. Pleura gorged with black, clotted blood. Stomach, intestines and mesentery highly congested. Large intestines much thickened, and contained small tubercles. Kidneys congested. Many small tubercles found in upper portions of lungs, some of which had softened. Immediate cause of death, thrombosis and embolism, caused by the acidity of blood from fermenting food. *Microscopic examinations :* Blood and contents of bowels found to contain the same vegetation as in the preceding case. Twenty-nine hogs have died since the morning of Nov. 1. Fifty-six in all have died from the lot of six hundred and twenty-four which were placed in the pens Oct. 4, just one month ago.

CASE X.   A large barrow, weighing 300 lbs., was taken with the " trip-hammer " pulsations in heart Nov. 2. He immediately refused food, became listless, gradually became more and more paralyzed, blind and deaf, and finally fell over and suddenly expired to-day, at 1 p. m., Nov. 4th. He had severe diarrhœa for about three weeks previous to death. Surface blue. Post-mortem at 3 p. m. Body still warm. Brain and meningeal vessels congested, with slight exudation of serum. Chest contained about one quart of clear serum. Pleura covered with a membrane of partially organized fibrin. Right lung gorged with black, clotted blood; gangrenous and softened. Left lung congested with black, clotted blood, but involved more recently than the right lung. Diaphragm gorged with black, clotted blood. Stomach highly congested. Mucous lining a dark red. Intestines and mesentery, and peritoneal membrane congested. Pleura congested. Liver gorged with black, clotted blood. Pericardium but slightly affected. Thrombus extending entirely through the heart and down the aorta. Death caused by thrombosis and embolism. Minute tubercles noticed in all parts of lungs. The blood contained the spores of the mycoderma acéti, and the contents of bowels, the vinegar and alcoholic yeast plants of fermenting grain.

CASE XI. *Symptoms before Death.* Diarrhœa set in on the 10th of Oct. At that time weight about 200 lbs. Has fallen away since that time so that now she weighs but 180 lbs. The "trip-hammer" pulsations of heart began yesterday afternoon, at which time she ceased to eat. Became listless; nose held to floor; reeled in walking; held head to one side, with one ear loped, frequently shaking the head, indicating ringing in the ears. These symptoms gradually grew worse, and at 12 m. to-day she fell over on the side, where she lay until she died, at 3 p. m., Nov. 4.—5 p. m. *Post-mortem.* Surface blue. Flesh still warm. Uterus and ovaries congested. Chest contained about four ounces of bloody serum. Lungs black with congestion. Blood-vessels completely filled with black, clotted blood. Upper portion of lungs filled with small tubercles. Heart, diaphragm and stomach not congested. Thrombus in heart. Stomach filled with slimy mucus and fermenting food. Intestines congested. Kidneys congested and filled with clots of blood. Death caused by embolism in lungs and kidneys. The microscopic examination discovered vinegar yeast spores in the blood, in numerous small masses; also this vegetation and the alcoholic yeast spores in the contents of the bowels.

CASE XII. Nov. 4, 7 p. m. First noticed with "trip-hammer" pulsations last evening. Died to-day at 12 m. Weight 200 lbs.; in fair condition. Had diarrhœa for over two weeks before death. Brain congested, with effusion of small quantity of serum. Chest contained about one pint of effused serum and clots of blood. Pleura highly inflamed. Left lung highly congested; a portion of right lung quite healthy, the balance involved in disease. Pericardium and external surface of heart congested. Kidneys quite healthy. Stomach slightly congested and filled with food. Intestines congested highly and gangrenous in spots. Death caused by embolism in lungs and intestines. The microscopic examination revealed the same yeast vegetation in blood and contents of bowels as were found in the preceding case.

Monday morning, 9 a. m., Nov. 5. Damp, cool, temperature 32° Fah. Temperature rose to 50° Fah. in afternoon. Eight fine hogs died last night, or since 6 p. m. last evening. Four of the eight were placed in the tank without examination. The other four were examined and the following are the results : —

Case XIII. Weight 180 lbs. Fair condition. Had been suffering with chronic diarrhœa, or consumption of bowels, for over two weeks. Died this morning at 7 a. m. In the last stages of its disease it discharged from nostrils and mouth a considerable quantity of mucus. This is common in all cases where the lungs are seriously involved. Lungs gorged with black, clotted blood, except a small portion around the edges. Color of lungs black, mottled with red and pink spots. Some small tubercles scattered all through the lungs. Pelves of kidneys and ureters gorged with clotted blood. Stomach gorged with blood near pyloric orifice. Filled with fermenting food and mucus. Intestines slightly congested. Large intestines thickened. Other organs healthy. Death caused by embolism in lungs and kidneys. Small masses of spores of mycoderma aceti were numerous in the blood, and the fermenting contents of bowels were filled with the same spores and those of alcoholic yeast (Saccharomyces).

Case XIV. Ten a. m., Nov. 5. Died this morning at 8 a. m. Still warm. Had diarrhœa for over two weeks before death. "Trip-hammer" pulsations first noticed day before yesterday, Nov. 3. Has been a more lingering case than usual. Weight

200 lbs. Meninges and sinuses of the brain full of blood; slight exudation of serum. Kidneys gorged with blood and pelves filled with clots. Uterus so gorged with black, clotted blood, that it is ruptured, discharging several ounces of clotted blood into the abdomen. This appears to have been the immediate cause of death. Stomach and intestines gorged with clotted blood and gangrenous in spots. Heart contained a thrombus. Liver quite healthy. Surface of body not blue. Lungs in fair condition, but slightly congested.

CASE XV. Nov. 5, 1 p. m. Died last night. Body not yet cold. Weight 160 lbs. "Trip-hammer" pulsations noticed yesterday. Surface very blue. Brain slightly congested, with small exudation of serum. Heart enlarged and softened, so that it tears easily. Surface covered with strings of partially organized fibrin. Pericardium contained about one pint of exuded serum. Pleural cavity contained about one quart of bloody serum. Pleura covered with shreds and small deposits of partially organized fibrin. Lungs gorged with black, clotted blood, softened and almost broken down. Liver quite natural. Kidneys healthy. Stomach and intestines slightly congested; large intestines thickened. Death caused by embolism in lungs and pericardium. Lungs contained small tubercular deposits.

CASE XVI. Nov. 5, 3 p. m. Died last night. First noticed sick yesterday. Surface very blue. Weight 200 lbs. Condition good. Had diarrhœa for nearly two weeks before death. Frothy, bloody mucus discharged from nostrils and mouth before death. Brain and membranes highly congested, with considerable effusion of bloody serum. Lungs gorged with black, clotted blood. Air cells filled with bloody mucus. Many small tubercles noticed in lung tissue. Chest contains about one quart of effused bloody serum. Heart gorged with clotted blood and enlarged. Pleura covered with shreds of partially organized fibrin. Kidneys slightly congested; an old abscess in each, about the size of a walnut. All other organs quite normal in appearance, except large intestines, which were thickened. In all the four cases examined to-day, the blood was found quite full of small masses of the spores of the mycoderma aceti, and the contents of bowels filled with the Micoderma and Saccharomyces.

CASE XVII. *Symptoms before death.* Had chronic diarrhœa for about three weeks. Was taken Nov. 5, early in the morning, with " trip-hammer " pulsations of heart. Ceased to eat ; became dumpish ; nose to floor ; reeled in walking ; head held to one side ; left ear loped ; shakes head frequently. At 4 p. m. fell over on side and began to twitch spasmodically, with trembling like ague. Breathing quick and labored ; pulse quick, short and spasmodic ; surface blue on under part of body ; warm, up to fever heat ; frothing at mouth and nostrils, froth bloody. These symptoms continued till 4 o'clock and 15 minutes, when, after a general tremor for a few moments, breathing ceased. Post-mortem immediately after death. Lungs gorged with black, clotted blood. Heart contained a thrombus. Meningeal vessels gorged with clotted blood. Stomach and large bowels thickened, and filled with mucus and fermenting food. The lungs contained many small tubercles. Death from embolism in the meningeal vessels and lungs.

CASE XVIII. Died at 3 p. m., Nov. 5. Post-mortem at 5.30 p. m. Flesh still warm. Weight 200 lbs. One lung filled with black, clotted blood ; the other quite healthy. Pelvis of kidneys filled with clotted blood ; so were also the ureters. Bladder contained about four ounces of blood. Stomach and large intestines congested and softened. Spleen gorged with clotted blood. Surface not blue. Death caused by embolism in one lung and kidneys. In this and the preceding case, the contents of bowels were filled with the spores of mycoderma aceti, and saccharomyces cerevisiæ, and the blood contained numerous small groups of the spores of the former vegetation.

CASE XIX. Nov. 6, 10 a. m. Two hogs have died since 6 p. m. last evening. Weight 160 lbs. Surface blue, and still warm. Pregnant. Pigs half grown. Lungs gorged with black, clotted blood and softened. Pleura contained about one quart of bloody serum. Kidneys quite healthy. Uterus congested. Stomach and large bowels congested ; of a cherry-red color on thin mucous surface. Urinary organs healthy. Death caused by embolism of lungs. A few small, tubercular deposits were found in lungs and walls of large intestines. Masses of vinegar yeast were found in blood, and this and alcoholic yeast found in great quantities in fermenting contents of bowels.

CASE XX. Nov. 6, 10 a. m. Died last night. Weight 160 lbs. Flesh still warm. Lungs but recently congested ; the clots in vessels not yet blackened; contain small quantity of exuded serum. Peritoneum congested and mottled with red and black. Slight congestion in one kidney; the other healthy. Stomach slightly congested and thickened ; contains inside many worms ; gall duct and gall bladder filled with worms : gall duct completely blocked up with them and clotted blood. Gall bladder filled with thick, black bile and worms. Liver, white and yellow, and softened so that it falls to pieces of its own weight. Death in this case caused by partial embolism in lungs, and stoppage of gall duct with worms. Worms from six to ten inches long. Counted thirty in the gall duct and gall bladder.

CASE XXI. Nov. 6, 4 p. m. Three died since 8 a. m. this morning. Flesh still warm. Surface not blue. Weight 150 lbs. Membrane of brain highly congested. Pleural cavity contained one pint of yellow serum, and pericardium four ounces of serum. Lungs gorged with clotted blood, except the lower lobes. External surface of heart gorged with black, clotted blood. Kidneys congested and their pelvis contained a small quantity of effused fluid blood. Pyloric end of the stomach congested and mucous membrane of a cherry-red color ; the balance of mucous surface of a pale lead color. Small intestines filled with worms, and the mucous lining filled with small white tubercles, the size of a wheat kernel, having a small cavity inside, and each one surrounded by a black ring, filled with black, clotted blood, thus : ⊖ ⊖ ⊖. Liver congested and gall-bladder filled with bile and blood. Death caused by embolism of brain, lungs, heart and kidneys. The tubercles in small intestines involved the entire thickness of their walls, so that when they were pulled out, holes were made through them the size of wheat kernels. The *microscopic examination* demonstrated the presence of large quantities of the spores of vinegar and alcoholic yeast vegetation in the fermenting matter in bowels, and numerous masses of vinegar yeast in the blood.

CASE XXII. Nov. 6, 5 p. m. Died 12 m. to-day. Flesh still warm. Weight 160 lbs. Surface blue. Brain gorged with black, clotted blood ; more so than any case before examined. Pleural cavity contains small quantity of bloody serum. Upper lobes of lungs gorged with black, clotted blood, and tissues partially broken down. Blood exuded in bronchial tubes. Lower portion of lungs quite good. Heart highly congested and covered with effused blood. Kidneys gorged with blood and ureters softened. Stomach congested. Liver white, bloodless and rotten. Gall bladder filled with bloody bile. Death caused by embolism of brain, heart, lungs and kidneys. The *microscopic examination* demonstrated the presence of the same vegetations in blood and contents of bowels, as were found in the previous case. Small tubercles were present in the lungs and small intestines.

CASE XXIII. Nov. 6, 6 p. m. Died since 12 m. to-day. Flesh still warm. Had chronic diarrhœa about three weeks before the " trip-hammer " pulsations of heart began yesterday. Surface very blue. Blood very black. Brain gorged with black, clotted blood. Pleural cavity contained one pint of bloody serum. Right lung gorged with black, clotted blood, and soft-ened so that it fell to pieces in handling. Left lung recently involved and gorged with blood. Small tubercles scattered throughout the lungs. Heart normal, except a long mass of fibrin extending through it, and some inches down the aorta. Liver gorged with black, clotted blood, and gall-bladder filled with bloody bile. Kidneys congested, and bladder contained bloody urine. Stomach congested and filled with yellow rice-water, matter and mucus. Large bowels thickened and congested. Digestive canal filled with yeast vegetation of acid and alcoholic types, and blood contained numerous masses of mycoderma aceti. Death caused by embolism of brain, lungs and liver.

CASE XXIV. 10 a. m. Died last night. Surface blue. Still warm. Membrane of brain congested, with small quantity of effused serum. Pleural cavity contained four ounces of ef-fused serum. Lungs gorged with black, clotted blood. Right lung only recently involved; the left of several days' standing.. Heart congested and filled with clotted blood. Liver slightly congested, and gall-bladder filled with a thick, tarry, black bile. Stomach congested near pyloric orifice. Kidneys congested. Large intestines congested and thickened. Tubercles (small) in lungs and small intestines, about the size of millet-seed. The same yeast vegetations were found in contents of bowels and blood as were present in previous cases. This hog had suffered with severe chronic diarrhœa for over three weeks before being taken with " trip-hammer " pulsations of heart. Died of em-bolism.

CASE XXV. Nov. 7, 10 a. m. *Symptoms before death.* Has had chronic diarrhœa for over three weeks. Was taken this morning with severe coughing, accompanied with " trip-hammer " pulsations of the heart. Pulsations 38 to 44 to the minute. Breathing labored. Nose held to the floor; scarcely notices anything; seems partially blind and deaf; reels in walking; breathing short and quick and 44 to the minute. Nov. 7, 3 p. m. Lying on side, unable to get up; respiration and pulsations the same as above; surface hot and feverish; eyes discharging water freely. Nov. 8, 10 a. m. Died during last night. Surface blue; flesh still warm. Brain and membranes congested, with small quantity of effused serum. Pleural cavity contains one pint of effused serum. Left lung filled with tubercles, and perfectly gorged with black, clotted blood; has the appearance of having been involved for two or three days. Right lung also gorged with clotted blood, but more recently involved. Heart somewhat congested, and contains a thrombus. Diaphragm congested. Stomach and large intestines congested, thickened and filled with fermenting matter and mucus. Kidneys congested and ureters filled with blood. All other organs quite healthy in appearance. Death from embolism in lungs. The contents of bowels and blood contain the same yeast vegetations as were found in the previous cases.

CASE XXVI. Nov. 8, 11 a. m. Large white hog, weighing 350 lbs. Died last night; still warm. Passed from bowels considerable blood before death. Had diarrhœa (or consumption of bowels) for over three weeks previous to fatal attack. " Trip-hammer " pulsations of heart began yesterday forenoon, and soon after was unable to walk or stand. Respirations and pulsations about forty to the minute. Post-mortem at 11 a. m., Nov. 8. Surface not blue. Brain and membranes congested. Pleural cavity contained one quart of effused bloody serum. Lungs filled with small tubercles. Right lung adhering to wall of chest, and filled with black, clotted blood. Left lung more recently involved, and filled with clotted blood, except the upper lobe, which was yet quite free from disease. Mesentery and large intestines filled with small tubercles, about the size of a pea, and all around them (each one) the tissues were gorged with black, clotted blood. Large intestines thickened. Stomach and bowels filled with fermenting food and mucus, and congested, the vessels being filled with black, clotted blood. Liver softened and white. Kidneys normal. Death caused by embolism of lungs and bowels. Blood contained an unusual quantity of small masses of spores of mycoderma aceti, and the contents of bowels and stomach were filled with the spores of mycoderma aceti and saccharomyces cerevisiæ.

CASE XXVII. Nov. 8, 12 m. Weight 200 lbs. Died last night. Still warm. Surface not blue. Had chronic diarrhœa for three weeks before the fatal attack. One lobe of brain congested; the other not involved. Lungs in healthy condition except a slight congestion in upper lobes. Heart contained a thrombus; otherwise healthy. Liver and kidneys in good condition. Stomach and intestines slightly congested, and large bowel thickened. Contain considerable fermenting food and yellow mucus. Muscles of abdomen — from navel back — gorged with black, clotted blood, and large masses of black, clotted blood, the size of a goose-egg, escaped from ruptured vessels, and lying between the muscles. Embolism in the abdominal muscles appears to have been the immediate cause of death; although the peritoneum had become more recently involved and no doubt hastened the result, as a secondary cause. The same vegetations were found in the blood and contents of bowels as in the previous cases.

CASE XXVIII. Nov. 8, 1 p. m. Weight 200 lbs. Died last night. Surface still warm. Surface blue. Had chronic diarrhœa, or consumption of bowels, for three weeks before death. "Trip-hammer" pulsations began yesterday morning. Brain highly congested. Pleural cavity contained one quart of effused, bloody serum. Fibrin deposited in shreds, and mammillated eminences on walls of pericardium and heart. Heart gorged with black, clotted blood and enlarged; contained a thrombus. Lungs contain many small tubercles, and gorged with black, clotted blood; one for many days and the other more recent.

Diaphragm congested. Kidneys congested. Liver normal. Stomach and intestines congested, and large intestine thickened. Whole intestinal track contains fermenting food and a yellowish mucus. Cause of death, embolism in lungs, heart and brain. The same vegetations found in the blood and contents of bowels in this case as in the previous ones.

CASE XXIX. Nov. 8, 1 p. m. Died last night. Surface blue. Weight 200 lbs. Had chronic diarrhœa for over three weeks before the fatal attack of Embolism. "Trip-hammer" pulsations began yesterday morning. Became soon so paralyzed that he could only walk a few steps at a time without falling. Ceased to eat; nose to floor, and head held to one side with one ear lopped. Shaking head frequently. Almost blind and deaf. Post-mortem at 1.30 p. m. Body still warm. Much bloated and has a foetid smell. Brain congested. Pleural cavity contains one pint of effused serum. Lungs partially gorged with black, clotted blood; contain many small tubercles. Liver gorged with black, clotted blood and softened. Spleen gorged with black, clotted blood and gangrenous. Heart softened and flabby, and contained a clot. Intestines highly congested, and black with clotted blood. Large intestines thickened. Stomach congested. Peritoneum black and gangrenous. Bladder congested and urine dark and muddy. Kidneys white and softened. Uterus gorged with clotted blood. Death caused by embolism in spleen, liver, intestines and lungs. The blood and contents of bowels contained the same yeast vegetations as were found in the preceding cases.

CASE XXX. Nov. 8, 3 p. m. Had chronic diarrhœa, or consumption of the bowels, for over two weeks previous to the fatal attack. "Trip-hammer" pulsations began yesterday forenoon. Died last night. Still warm. Surface blue. Brain and its membranes congested. Pleural cavity contained one pint of clear serum. Walls of pericardium and heart covered with shreds and mammillàted deposits of fibrin. Lungs gorged with black, clotted blood. Air cells filled with bloody, frothy mucus. Lung tissues softened in places and contained many small tubercles. Heart flabby and softened, and contained a thrombus. Diaphragm gorged with black, clotted blood. Kidneys congested, and pelves of contained small clots of blood. Ureters congested. Stomach congested and thickened. Large intestines thickened and congested; contain fermenting food and yellowish mucus. Blood and contents of bowels filled with the same yeast vegetations as were found in the previous cases. Death caused by embolism in lungs, diaphragm and kidneys.

CASE XXXI. Nov. 8, 4 p. m. Had chronic diarrhœa for three weeks before the fatal attack. "Trip-hammer" pulsations began early yesterday morning. Died last night. Body still warm; surface not blue. Weight 250 lbs. Brain congested and also its membranes. Pleural cavity contained one pint of bloody serum. Pericardium filled with bloody serum. Lungs gorged with black, clotted blood, except the upper lobes, which were still quite healthy. Filled with small tubercles. Heart filled with black, clotted blood. Stomach and intestines highly congested. Liver and spleen congested. Kidneys congested and pelves filled with small clots of black blood. Blood and contents of bowels contained the same yeast vegetations as were found in the preceding cases. Death caused by embolism in lungs, liver, spleen and kidneys.

CASE XXXII. Nov. 8, 5 p. m. Had chronic diarrhœa for over two weeks before death. "Trip-hammer" pulsations began yesterday forenoon. Died last night. Surface blue. Brain and membranes congested, and contained about two ounces of effused serum. Lungs filled with black, clotted blood. Pleural cavity contained one quart of bloody serum. Lung tissue contains many small tubercles the size of a millet seed, some of which were softened. Heart contained a thrombus. Pericardium contained about six ounces of bloody serum. Stomach and large intestines congested and thickened. Kidneys gorged with black, clotted blood. Blood and contents of bowels unusually filled with the yeast vegetations found in the previous cases. Death caused by embolism in lungs, brain and kidneys.

CASE XXXIII. Nov. 9. Three hogs died last night. All had diarrhœa, or consumption of bowels, for over three weeks before death. "Trip-hammer" pulsations began in all of them yesterday forenoon. The first examined weighed 150 lbs. Flesh still warm. Surface not blue. Brain and its membranes congested. Small effusion of serum in pleural cavity. Left lung and upper lobe of right gorged with black, clotted blood. Lower lobe of right lung quite good. Lungs contain many small tubercles, the size of millet seed. Heart congested, and auricles and ventricles filled full of black, clotted blood. Kidneys congested and pelves and ureters contain small clots of effused blood. Liver congested and of a brown-black, inky color, and softened. Large intestines thickened and contain a jelly-like mucus, and fermenting food. Death caused by embolism of lungs, liver and kidneys, with thrombus in heart. Blood and bowels contain the same yeast vegetations as were found in all the previous cases.

CASE XXXIV. Nov. 10. Last night was cold, cloudy and windy. Snow fell just enough to cover the surface. Temperature from 35° to 40° Fah. Rained slightly during the day. Seven hogs died since yesterday morning at 10 a. m. All had chronic diarrhœa or consumption of bowels for over three weeks before death. The "trip-hammer" pulsations began in all of them from twelve to fourteen hours before the fatal termination. The surface was blue in all of them. A post-mortem was made only in one of these cases. At 4 p. m., flesh still warm; surface blue. Brain and membranes badly congested. Pleural cavity contained about one pint of effused serum, and its walls were highly congested. Lungs perfectly gorged with black, clotted blood, and softened. Contain many small tubercles. Heart congested and contained a thrombus. Kidneys congested in upper portions. Liver congested. Large intestines congested and walls thickened. Blood and contents of bowels contained the same yeast vegetations as were found in the previous cases. Death caused by embolism in lungs.

CASE XXXV. Nov. 11, 10 a. m. Eight hogs died since 10 a. m. yesterday. Weather cool, wet and cloudy. Temperature 40° to 45° Fah. Made post-mortem of only one of the eight. Surfaces of all were blue. All had suffered with consumption of bowels for over three weeks. " Trip-hammer " pulsations began in all about twelve hours before death. Weight of one examined : 180 lbs. Flesh still warm. Brain and membranes congested, resulting in small effusion of serum. Pleural cavity contained about one quart of effused, bloody serum. Walls covered with deposits of fibrin and clots of blood. Lungs gorged with black, clotted blood, save the edges of right lung. Contained many small tubercles. Kidneys gorged with black blood, and pelves and ureters filled with clots. Bladder filled with bloody urine. Liver congested. Large intestines thickened and congested, and partly filled with slimy mucus and fermenting food. Blood and contents of bowels unusually full of the yeast vegetations found in previous cases. Death caused by embolism of lungs, heart and kidneys.

CASE XXXVI. Nov. 12. Three hogs have died since 10 a. m. yesterday. All had had chronic diarrhœa for over three weeks. The "trip-hammer" pulsations began in all of them early yesterday morning. A post-mortem was made in only one of the cases. This was a small spotted sow; weight 130 lbs. Brain and membranes congested. Lungs but slightly congested. Kidneys normal. Heart filled with clotted blood. Stomach highly congested and mucous surface of a mahogany-red color. Intestines congested and gorged with black, clotted blood; walls thickened, and large bowels filled with effused blood and partially organized fibrin. Upper portion of small intestines ulcerated. Intestines perfectly closed up with pus, blood and fibrin. Walls of bowels contain many small tubercles. Death caused by ulceration and embolism of bowels.

CASE XXXVII. Nov. 13. Six hogs have died since yesterday at 4 p. m. Post-mortems were made of five of these. All had chronic diarrhœa for over three weeks before death. Large sow, weight 220 lbs. In fine condition. Flesh still warm. Brain and membranes slightly congested. No effusion. Pleural cavity contained about one pint of effused serum. Walls of cavity covered with partially organized fibrin, in eminences and shreds. Lungs gorged with black, clotted blood, and upper lobes contain many small tubercles. Heart filled with firm clots and enlarged. A fatty tumor, the size of a hen's egg, in auricle. Liver whitish and softened. Kidneys highly congested, and pelves and ureters gorged with clotted blood. Stomach and large intestines congested and thickened, and contained slimy mucus and fermenting food. Chest and abdomen give off a fœtid odor. Blood and contents of bowels unusually full of the yeast vegetations found in previous cases. Death caused by thrombosis of heart, and embolism in lungs and kidneys.

CASE XXXVIII. Nov. 13. Died last night. Weight 150 lbs. Surface not blue. Brain and membranes slightly congested; no effusion. Pleural cavity contains about eight ounces of effused, bloody serum. Lungs gorged with black, clotted blood, except a small portion of lung on right side. Heart filled with black clots. Kidneys congested and pelves and ureters filled with black, clotted blood. Liver softened and of a grayish-white color. Gall-bladder filled with black, clotted blood and bile. Large intestines congested and thickened, and contain a few small tubercles. Filled with slimy mucus and fermenting food. Blood and contents of bowels contain the same yeast vegetations found in all the previous cases. Immediate cause of death, embolism of lungs and thrombosis.

CASE XXXIX. Nov. 13. Died early this morning. Weight 180 lbs. Surface not blue. In fair condition. Membranes of brain gorged with clotted blood, resulting in a considerable effusion of bloody serum. Pleural cavity contained from twelve to sixteen ounces of effused bloody serum. Old disease in left lung; had become hepatized, hardened and gangrenous. The other is more recently affected, and both are gorged with black, clotted blood. Air cells filled with frothy, bloody mucus. Both lungs contained many small tubercles. Heart congested and filled with black blood clots. Kidneys gorged with black, clotted blood, and pelves and ureters filled with clotted blood. Stomach perfectly white inside; bloodless. Large intestines congested and thickened, and filled with slimy mucus and fermenting food. Liver congested. Uterus highly congested. Blood and digestive organs filled with the same yeast vegetations as were found in previous cases. Immediate cause of death, embolism of lungs and heart clots.

CASE XL. Nov. 13. Died early this morning. Weight 170 lbs. Surface not blue. Brain and membranes highly congested, and filled with black blood, resulting in effusion of two or three ounces of bloody serum. Pleural cavity contains ten to twelve ounces of effused, bloody serum. Right lung softened, suppurating and adhering to walls of chest. Other lung gorged with black blood, except the superior portion. Both contain many small tubercles. Heart congested, softened and filled with black blood clots. Liver gorged with black, clotted blood; gall-bladder filled with blood and bile. Stomach and intestines congested; large intestines thickened, and contain slimy mucus and fermenting food. Kidneys gorged with black, clotted blood; pelves and ureters contain blood clots; urine is bloody. Blood and contents of bowels contain the same yeast vegetations as were found in all the previous cases. Immediate cause of death, embolism in lungs, liver and kidneys, and heart clots.

CASE XLI. Nov. 13. Large sow. Weight 250 lbs. In fair condition. Surface blue. Died late last night. Brain and membranes gorged with clotted blood, resulting in the effusion of three or four ounces of bloody serum. Pleural cavity contains about one quart of effused, bloody serum. Walls covered with deposits of partially organized fibrin. Lungs gorged with black, clotted blood. Contain small tubercles in upper portions. Heart highly congested and auricles filled with black, clotted blood. Ventricles contain masses of fatty jelly. Liver highly congested. Stomach highly congested and of a dark color. Intestines highly congested and contain bloody mucus. Kidneys slightly congested. Pregnant. Pigs nearly full-grown; eight in all. Uterus gorged with black, clotted blood. Blood and intestines contain the same yeast vegetations as were found in all the preceding cases. Immediate cause of death, embolism of lungs, brain and intestines, and heart partly filled with tough clots.

CASE XLII. Nov. 14, 10 a. m. Four have died since 10 a. m. yesterday. The surfaces of all were blue. They all had had chronic diarrhœa, or consumption of bowels, for over three weeks. The "trip-hammer" pulsations began in all of them night before last and early yesterday morning. Only one of these was examined. Flesh cold. Brain and membranes highly congested. Pleural cavity contained from twelve to fourteen ounces of effused, bloody serum. Lungs gorged with black, clotted blood; contain a few tubercles. Heart filled with black, clotted blood. Stomach and intestines congested; large intestines thickened, and filled with slimy mucus and fermenting food. Kidneys gorged with black, clotted blood, and pelves and ureters contain blood. Same yeast vegetations found in blood and contents of bowels as were found in the preceding cases. Immediate cause of death, embolism of lungs and kidneys, and heart filled with tough blood clots.

CASE XLIII. Nov. 15, 10 a. m. Seven hogs died since yesterday at 10 a. m. All had chronic diarrhœa for over three weeks. The "trip-hammer" pulsations began in all of them from ten to fourteen hours before death. Post-mortem examinations were made of six of these seven. Died yesterday. Flesh cold. Surface cold. Weight 140 lbs. Fair condition. Brain and membranes highly congested, causing considerable effusion of bloody serum. Lungs gorged with black, clotted blood, and walls of chest covered with deposited fibrin, and clots of blood. Cavity contains six ounces of effused, bloody serum. Stomach and large intestines congested and thickened; the latter filled with slimy mucus and fermenting food. Heart filled with tough clots. Kidneys highly congested; their pelves and the ureters contain clots of blood. Urine bloody. Liver congested and softened. Blood and contents of bowels contain the same yeast vegetations as were found in all the preceding cases. Immediate cause of death, embolism of lungs, brain and kidneys and tough heart clots.

CASE XLIV. Nov. 15. Died last night. Weight 160 lbs. Flesh warm. Surface not blue. Brain and membranes congested, resulting in effusion of about one ounce of serum. One lung badly gorged with black, clotted blood, the other one partially involved. Chest contains about four ounces of effused, bloody serum. Lungs contain many small tubercles. Stomach highly congested; also intestines; large intestines filled with slimy mucus and fermenting food, and walls of, thickened. Blood and contents of bowels contain the same yeast vegetations as were found in all the preceding cases. Immediate cause of death, embolism in lungs and brain.

Case XLV. Nov. 15. Died last night. Flesh still warm. Surface not blue. Brain congested, with effusion of small quantity of serum. Lungs gorged with black, clotted blood, except in upper lobes, with effusion of about four ounces of serum. Liver whitish-gray, and softened. Kidneys congested. Stomach and intestines congested; large bowels thickened, and filled with slimy mucus and fermenting food. Heart flabby and filled with clots. Blood contained many small masses of the spores of mycoderma aceti, and the contents of bowels the same vegetation, and a large quantity of the spores of the saccharomyces cerevisiæ. Immediate cause of death, embolism of lungs and brain.

Case XLVI. Nov. 15. Died last night. Weight 160 lbs. Surface blue. Flesh still warm. Brain highly congested, with effusion of bloody serum on surface. Pleura highly congested. Lungs gorged with black, clotted blood; contain many small tubercles. · Liver grayish-white and softened. Stomach congested and filled with a yellow slime. Intestines congested and blackened, vessels being gorged with dark blood. Kidneys gorged with black blood, and clots of blood in pelves of, and in ureters. Same yeast vegetations found in the blood and bowels in this case as in the preceding ones. Immediate cause of death, embolism of lungs, intestines, kidneys and brain.

Case XLVII. Nov. 15. Died last night. Weight 170 lbs. Flesh still warm. Surface still blue. Brain and membranes highly congested, with effusion of about one ounce of serum. Lungs partially gorged with black, clotted blood; serous lining of chest gorged with blood, and covered with effused, clotted blood and lymph. Liver congested and blackened on lower surface. Heart congested and filled with firm clots. Stomach and intestines highly congested; lower bowels thickened and filled with slimy mucus and fermenting food. Kidneys highly congested, pelves and ureters filled with clotted blood. Urine bloody. Same yeast vegetations found in the blood and contents of bowels as were found in the preceding cases. Immediate cause of death : embolism of lungs, kidneys, brain and liver.

CASE XLVIII. Nov. 15. Small hog. Weight 90 lbs. Surface blue. Died yesterday. Brain congested and effusion on surface. Cavity of chest contained from twelve to fourteen ounces of effused serum. Walls covered with partially organized fibrin in shreds and small eminences. Lungs full of tubercles and gorged with black, clotted blood. Liver gorged with blood, black and softened. Stomach filled with water. Intestines highly congested ; lower portion thickened and filled with slimy mucus and fermenting food. Kidneys congested. Blood and contents of bowels unusually full of yeast vegetations, such as found in the previous cases. Immediate cause of death : embolism of lungs, liver and brain.

CASE XLIX. Nov. 16, 4 p. m. Seven hogs have died since 10 a. m. yesterday. Post mortems were made of six of them. All had suffered with chronic diarrhœa, or consumption of bowels, for over three weeks. The " trip-hammer " pulsations began in all from ten to fourteen hours before death. Died last night. Surface not blue. Weight 190 lbs. Brain highly congested, with considerable surface effusion. Chest and abdominal cavity contained from two to four quarts of effused, black blood and serum. Lungs gorged with black, clotted blood, and filled with small tubercles. Liver white, softened, enlarged. Falls in pieces on handling. Kidneys gorged with blood and softened. Blood in abdominal cavity comes from bursting of ureters ; that in chest from effusion. Heart gorged with black, clotted blood and softened. Stomach and intestines highly congested and softened. Lower bowels thickened. Immediate cause of death : embolism of lungs, liver, kidneys, stomach, bowels and heart. Blood and contents of bowels unusually full of the yeast vegetations found in previous cases.

Case L. Nov. 16. Died last night. Weight 150 lbs. Surface blue. Brain and membranes slightly congested. No effusion. Lungs gorged with black, clotted blood, resulting in about two ounces of effused serum. Heart filled with tough clots. Kidneys highly congested and pelvis and ureters filled with clotted blood. Ovaries filled with clotted blood. Liver normal. Stomach and intestines congested ; lower bowels thickened and filled with slimy mucus and fermenting food. Lungs contain a few small tubercles. Blood and contents of bowels contain the same kind of yeast vegetations as were found in the previous cases. Immediate cause of death : embolism in lungs, kidneys and ovaries.

Case LI. Nov. 16. Died last night. Weight 200 lbs. Surface blue. Brain and membranes congested. No effusion. Chest contains four ounces of effused serum. Lungs gorged with black, clotted blood ; contain small tubercles. Liver gorged with black blood, and so softened that it falls in pieces on handling. Intestines black, from blood-vessels being gorged with dark, clotted blood. Stomach in same condition. Large bowels thickened and filled with slimy mucus and fermenting food. Uterus congested, and contained half a dozen half-grown pigs. Heart filled with dark blood clots, and softened. All the organs in chest and abdomen emitted a very fœtid odor from partial decay, or perhaps gangrene before death. Blood contained the same yeast vegetations as were found in the preceding cases. Immediate cause of death, extensive embolism of all the organs of chest and abdomen.

Case LII. Nov. 16. Died last night. Weight 160 lbs. Surface blue. Brain and membranes congested, but no effusion. Chest contained four ounces of effused serum. Lungs gorged with black, clotted blood, in all except the extreme upper portions ; contain many small tubercles. Liver normal. Heart softened and filled with clotted blood. Kidneys and ureters highly congested. Stomach and intestines highly congested, and filled with yellow, slimy mucus and fermenting food. Large bowels thickened. Blood contained the mycoderma aceti, and the stomach and bowels, this fungus and the saccharomyces cerevisiæ. Immediate cause of death : embolism of lungs and bowels.

CASE LIII. Nov. 16. Died to-day. Weight 190 lbs. Surface not blue. Flesh still warm. Brain and membranes congested, with effusion of about one ounce of serum. Lungs in fair condition ; contain a few small tubercles. Heart soft, flabby and filled with clots. Kidneys highly congested ; pelves of, and ureters filled with clotted blood. Stomach and intestines congested ; lower bowels thickened, and filled with slimy matter and fermenting food. Blood and contents of bowels contained the same yeast vegetations as were found in the cases previously examined. Immediate cause of death : congestion of brain and embolism of kidneys.

CASE LIV. Nov. 16. Died to-day. Weight 180 lbs. Flesh still warm. Brain and membranes congested, but no effusion. Chest contained one pint of effused, bloody serum. Lungs filled with black, clotted blood, and contain many small tubercles. Heart soft, flabby and filled with clots. Stomach and intestines highly congested ; large bowels thickened and filled with slimy mucus and fermenting food. Kidneys gorged with black, clotted blood ; pelves of, and ureters filled with clots, and urine bloody. Pregnant. Pigs nearly grown. Blood contained the same yeast vegetations as were found in the preceding cases. Immediate cause of death, embolism of lungs and kidneys.

CASE LV. Nov. 17, 10 a. m. Two hogs have died since 4 p. m. yesterday. There is an evident improvement in the hogs in the pen. All appear more lively and feed better, and the diarrhœa is less. Post mortems were made of both the hogs that have died since 4 p. m. yesterday. They both had diarrhœa for over three weeks. The "trip-hammer" pulsations began in them about twelve hours before death. Weight 200 lbs. Surface blue. Flesh warm. Brain and membranes badly congested, with effusion of about two ounces of bloody serum. Chest walls highly congested, and cavity of chest contained one pint of effused bloody serum. Lungs gorged with black, clotted blood and softened. Contained many small tubercles, the size of millet seeds. Kidneys gorged with black, clotted blood, and pelves of, and ureters filled with clots. Ureters ruptured, and clotted blood discharged into the abdominal cavity. Urine full of mucus. Stomach and intestines highly congested; lower bowels thickened and filled with slimy mucus and fermenting food. Blood and contents of bowels unusually filled with the yeast vegetations found in the previous cases. Immediate cause of death: embolism of lungs, kidneys and brain.

Case LVI. Nov. 17. Died last night. Weight 150 lbs. Surface not blue. Brain and membranes congested; no effusion. Lungs only partially gorged with blood. Contain small tubercles. Cavity of chest contained one pint of effused, bloody serum. Pericardium contained about four ounces of effused bloody serum. Liver congested and softened. Kidneys congested. Stomach filled with yellow, slimy fluid. Several small cauliflower excrescences on mucous surface of stomach, the size of a hickory nut. Excrescences of a deep chrome-yellow color, and are made up of enlarged follicles. It is from these that the yellow matter found in the stomach emanated. Intestines congested; large bowels thickened and filled with slimy mucus and fermenting food. Blood and contents of bowels contained the same yeast vegetations found in the preceding cases. Immediate cause of death: embolism of lungs, heart and liver.

Case LVII. Nov. 18, 11 a. m. Two hogs have died since

10 a. m. yesterday. Both had chronic diarrhœa for nearly four weeks. The "trip-hammer" pulsations began in each about twelve hours before death. Both examined. Weight 200 lbs. Lungs gorged with black, clotted blood, and contain small tubercles. Kidneys gorged with black, clotted blood ; pelves of, and ureters filled with clots. Heart filled with clots. Stomach and intestines congested ; lower bowel thickened and filled with a jelly-like mucus and fermenting food. Immediate cause of death, embolism of lungs and kidneys.

CASE LVIII. Nov. 18. Weight 200 lbs. Brain and membranes congested and covered with effused bloody serum. Right lung broken down, except small portion of upper lobe, which is filled with tubercles. Left lung filled with black, clotted blood, and contained many small tubercles. Liver congested. Large intestines thickened and filled with a jelly-like mucus and fermenting food. Kidneys congested. Blood and contents of bowels unusually full of the yeast vegetations found in previous cases. Immediate cause of death, embolism of left lung and brain. This hog had had a severe cough for several weeks. The cavity formed by the broken-down right lung was partially filled with pus. Although this hog died of embolism, if this had not occurred it would have soon died of consumption, as one lung was almost entirely broken down.

Nov. 19. Three hogs have died since the 17th. Did not make post-mortem examinations of them. They had had chronic diarrhœa for about four weeks. Both had "trip-hammer" pulsations of heart for some hours before death.

Nov. 28. The hogs have ceased dying in the pens of 624 which were penned on the 4th of October. Only six have died since the 19th. All appear healthy and vigorous. Did not make post-mortem examinations of these six. The hogs began to die in pen the 20th of October, just sixteen days after having been put on slop, and continued to die up to Nov. 28;

about eight weeks after being placed on this food. The deaths continued through a period of thirty-nine days. During this period 154 died in the pen of 624. The average death rate per day during this period was 3.95. The first fifteen days it was five per day; the next eleven days, $6\frac{4}{11}$ per day, and the last eleven days, $1\frac{9}{11}$ per day. Percentage that died, $24\frac{68}{100}$. Post mortems were made in fifty-eight cases, taken indiscriminately.

Oct. 25, 1858. Another lot of 404 hogs, just driven in from the surrounding country, where they were purchased from farmers, were placed in another pen, and put upon the slop from the whiskey distillery. This slop is the residue from the steam stills, after distilling off the "high wines." It is always very sour, from the presence of acetic acid (vinegar), and is filled with alcoholic and vinegar yeast (saccharomyces cerevisiæ, and mycoderma aceti).

These hogs were all in the finest and healthiest condition, and would average in weight 170 to 180 lbs. each.

By way of explanation, I will here state that each bushel of corn produces about forty gallons of slop. Each gallon of slop contains about four drams of acetic acid. Of the $78\frac{66}{100}$ per cent. of nutritious matter in corn, all is used up in the process of whiskey-making (alcoholic fermentation), but $12\frac{66}{100}$ per cent., which is itself partially decomposed. This renders the slop worth for fattening purposes, less than $\frac{1}{3}$ or $\frac{1}{4}$ that of the grain. When the hogs are on full feed, each hog is allowed eight gallons per day. During the first eight weeks, however, the new hogs are kept on short feed, and are only allowed five gallons each per day.

Oct. 25. Fed ravenously. Wanted more feed than was allowed them.

Oct. 26 and 27. Feeding ravenously. Very active; squealing and tearing about the pen; fighting and very uneasy.

Oct. 28. Beginning to get costive, and bloating up with wind. Still ravenous for more food; very uneasy.

Oct. 29. Becoming quite constipated, and very much bloated. Stools hard and becoming darker and more scanty.

Oct. 30 and 31. Constipation increasing, and bloating from flatulence much worse. Hogs getting more quiet, but still very hungry for more slop. Passing wind often.

Nov. 1–8. Hogs all very much constipated and disturbed with flatulence. Stools scanty, seldom, dark-colored and hard. Still hungry, but less ravenous for food.

Nov. 9–13. Constipation giving way to spurts of diarrhœa, with great quantities of wind. Hogs seem more or less dizzy, reeling in the walk sometimes, and less ravenous for food. Up to this date, four hogs have become so injured in the pen by fighting that they have been slaughtered. This leaves 400 in the pen.

CASE LIX. Nov. 13, 3½ p. m., the first hog died. Weighed 133 lbs. On making post-mortem examination, found all the organs healthy except the brain, which was gorged with clotted blood, with a blood-vessel broken. Died suddenly by the feeding-trough. Immediate cause of death, embolism of brain. Lungs contained no tubercular deposits. Bowels were filled with fermenting food. Post mortem was made immediately after death, and the blood was found clotted and thickened in heart, and in all the large vessels.

Nov. 14–18. Diarrhœa in all the hogs. Passages watery, numerous, and accompanied with a great amount of carbonic acid gas. Stools large and very light-colored; full of alcoholic and vinegar yeast vegetations.

CASE LX. Nov. 19. Hog died at 12½ p. m. Had been sick about 36 hours with "trip-hammer" pulsations, during which time it would eat nothing; nose held to floor, and reeled in walking. Partially deaf and blind, and partially paralyzed, especially in all the posterior parts of the body. Had chronic diarrhœa for about two weeks and a half before death. One lung was found filled with black, clotted blood; the other filled with bright red blood partially clotted. Heart filled with long strings and lumps (thrombi) of partially organized white fibrin. Pleura congested and inflamed. Kidneys congested and pelves of, contain clotted blood. Bladder highly congested. Liver healthy in appearance. Stomach filled with bloody serous fluid. Mucous membrane towards the pyloric orifice highly congested and inflamed. Duodenum in the same condition as pyloric end of the stomach. Intestines highly congested and thickened, especially the colon. Brain congested, with slight effusion of bloody serum. Blood and contents of digestive organs filled with yeast vegetation, the former containing vinegar yeast only, and the latter vinegar and alcoholic yeast. Immediate cause of death : thrombi in heart and embolism of lungs, kidneys, stomach and intestines.

CASE LXI. Nov. 20. Hog died last night. Has been weak and feeble ever since it was placed in pen. Never eaten at all well. Had been very costive up to within a week, when diarrhœa set in. Cavity of chest contained from two to three quarts of serum ; filled with masses of clear gelatine, like jelly. Lungs partially filled with black, clotted blood. Pericardium filled with serum. Stomach quite empty, and walls filled with dark, clotted blood. Whole intestinal canal congested and partially gangrenous ; contained many long tape-worms, firmly attached to walls of, and at the points of attachment were small white tubercles, the size of a pea. Brain congested, with considerable effusion of serum. Liver, spleen and kidneys healthy. Immediate cause of death, embolism of lungs, intestines, stomach and brain. One peculiarity in this case was the large effusion of serum and the aggregation of gelatine in partially organized masses in cavity of chest. The same yeast vegetations were found abundantly in the blood and contents of bowels in this case, that were found in the cases heretofore examined.

CASE LXII. Nov. 21. One hog died last night of hog-cholera. It had suffered with chronic diarrhœa for about two weeks previous to death. The "trip-hammer" pulsations began about fourteen hours before death. Lungs filled with black, clotted blood, and cavity of chest contained about one pint of effused serum. Long thrombi, or white fibrinous clots extended through the heart and into the large vessels leading from it. Stomach and large intestines congested and vessels of, filled with clotted blood. Small tubercles were found in walls of small intestines and upper lobes of lungs. Brain congested with effusion of small amount of serum. Other organs comparatively healthy. Blood contained the spores of mycoderma aceti, and the contents of bowels, the mycoderma aceti and saccharomyces cerevisiæ. Immediate cause of death, thrombus of heart and embolism of lungs, brain and intestinal walls.

CASE LXIII. Nov. 22. A small barrow, weighing 130 lbs. Died last night of Hog Cholera. Sudden asphyxia the immediate cause of death. "Trip-hammer" pulsations began only a few hours before death. Surface blue. Lungs gorged with black, clotted blood. Heart filled with thrombi extending through it into the large, out-going vessels. Stomach and large intestines congested. Other organs apparently healthy. Blood and contents of bowels contained the same yeast vegetations as were found in the previous cases. Immediate cause of death, thrombosis of heart and embolism of lungs.

Nov. 23. Three hogs died last night of Hog Cholera. All these had had chronic diarrhœa for about two weeks and a half. "Trip-hammer" pulsations began in them all during the afternoon of the 22d.

CASE LXIV. (1.) Sow, weighing 130 lbs. Surface white. Lungs partially congested and filled with black, clotted blood in lower lobes. Stomach and large intestines congested and thickened. Contents of a bright yellow color, thin and gelatinous. Heart contained several thrombi. Other organs apparently healthy. The same yeast vegetations found in this as in previous cases. Immediate cause of death, thrombosis and embolism.

CASE LXV. (2.) Barrow; weight 120 lbs. Surface blue. Lungs highly congested and filled with black, clotted blood. Heart congested and contained small thrombi. Cavity of chest contained about one pint of effused serum. Stomach and larger intestines congested and thickened, and filled with thin, yellow, slimy matters. Other organs healthy. Small tubercles in lungs. Blood and contents of bowels contained the same yeast vegetations as were found in the previous cases. Immediate cause of death, thrombosis and embolism.

CASE LXVI. (3.) Barrow; weight 130 lbs. Surface blue. Lungs gorged with black, clotted blood and filled with small tubercles. Cavity of chest contained about one pint of effused serum. Heart filled with thrombi and loose clots. Liver blackened with clotted blood. Stomach and large intestines congested and thickened, and filled with thin, yellow, slimy, fomenting matter. Kidneys congested. Same yeast vegetations found in blood and contents of bowels as were found in previous cases. Immediate cause of death, thrombi in heart, and embolism in lungs, liver and intestinal walls.

CASE LXVII. Nov. 24. Eight hogs have died since yesterday 12 m. (1.) Small hog, weighing 100 lbs. Surface blue. Lungs highly congested and filled with black, clotted blood. Contain many small tubercles. In cavity of chest was found about one pint of effused bloody serum. Pleura congested. Heart filled with loose clots and several thrombi. Pericardium contained about two ounces of serum. Stomach highly congested, empty and corrugated. Intestines congested and nearly empty. Brain congested, and membranes reddened, with slight effusion. Blood and bowels contained same yeast vegetations as were found in previous cases. Immediate cause of death, thrombosis and embolism.

Case LXVIII. (2.) Small hog; weight about 100 lbs. Surface blue. Had chronic diarrhœa for about two weeks before death. "Trip-hammer" pulsations set in twelve hours before death. Lungs gorged with black, clotted blood, and cavity of chest contained about one half pint of effused serum. Both lungs contained many small tubercles. Heart filled with loose clots and several thrombi extending through it into the outgoing vessels. Stomach and large intestines congested, and walls thickened. Contents slimy and yeasty. Liver congested and gorged with black blood. Other organs comparatively healthy. Blood contained numerous groups of mycoderma aceti and contents of bowels the same vegetation with alcoholic yeast. Immediate cause of death, thrombosis of heart and embolism of lungs and liver.

Case LXIX. (3.) Small hog; weight about 75 lbs. Quite thin from severe chronic diarrhœa for over two weeks. Trip-hammer pulsations began fourteen hours before death. Became paralyzed and unable to stand; soon after trip-hammer pulsations began. Surface blue. Lungs gorged with black, clotted blood and contained many small tubercles. Pleural cavity contained about four ounces of effused serum. Heart filled with clotted blood and contained several long thrombi, extending through it into the outgoing vessels. Brain congested, and cranial cavity contained about one ounce of effused serum. Blood and contents of bowels contained the same yeast vegetations as were found in the previous case. Immediate cause of death, thrombosis of heart and embolism of lungs and brain.

Case LXX. (4.) Barrow; weight 135 lbs. Good condition. Surface blue. Had chronic diarrhœa about one week before death. Trip-hammer began about twelve hours before life became extinct. Lungs gorged with black, clotted blood. Heart contained clots and thrombi. Pericardium congested, resulting in effusion of two ounces of serum. Cavity of chest contained about six (6) ounces of serum. Could detect no tubercles in lungs. Stomach and intestines congested and blackened, and contents slimy and yeasty. Other organs comparatively healthy. Blood and contents of bowels contained the same yeast vegetations as were found in the previous cases. Immediate cause of death, thrombosis and embolism.

CASE LXXI. (5.) Barrow; weight 120 lbs. Had chronic diarrhœa for about two weeks before death. Trip-hammer pulsations began about sixteen hours before life ceased. Surface blue. Lungs gorged with black, clotted blood and filled with small tubercles. Cavity of chest contained about one quart of effused bloody serum. Liver gorged with black, clotted blood and softened. Peritoneal cavity contained about one quart of effused bloody serum. Heart filled with clots and thrombi. Large intestines thickened and filled with slimy fermenting matter. Brain congested. Blood and contents of bowels contained the same yeast vegetations found in previous cases. Immediate cause of death, thrombosis and embolism.

CASE LXXII. (6.) Weight 140 lbs. Surface blue. Had chronic diarrhœa for about three weeks. Trip-hammer pulsations began about fourteen hours before death. Lungs gorged with black, clotted blood and contained many small tubercles. Cavity of chest contained about one pint of effused serum. Heart filled with clots and thrombi. Pericardium congested and containing about two (2) ounces of effused serum. Liver gorged with black, clotted blood. Spleen in the same condition. Kidneys gorged with clotted blood and blackened. Stomach and large intestines congested and thickened; contents of, slimy, yeasty and small. Blood and contents of bowels contained the same yeast vegetations as were found in the previous cases. Immediate cause of death, thrombosis and embolism.

CASE LXXIII. (7.) Weight 160 lbs. Surface blue. Had chronic diarrhœa for about three weeks. Trip-hammer pulsations began about eighteen hours before death. Lungs gorged with black, clotted blood and contained many small tubercles. Cavity of chest contained about one pint of effused serum. Heart contained three large thrombi. Pericardium contained about one ounce of effused serum. Stomach and large intestines congested and thickened, and the latter contained quite a quantity of jelly-like mucus with fermenting food. Kidneys congested and pelves of, contain clots of blood. Brain congested. Blood and contents of bowels contained the same yeast vegetations as were found in all the previously examined cases. Immediate cause of death, thrombosis and embolism.

CASE LXXIV. (8.) Weight 150 lbs. Fair condition. Surface blue. Had chronic diarrhœa for about two weeks. Trip-hammer pulsations began about sixteen hours before death. Lungs gorged with black, clotted blood and contained a few small tubercles. Cavity of chest contained about one pint of effused bloody serum. Heart filled with clots and several small thrombi. Liver gorged with clotted blood. Stomach and large bowels congested, and the latter thickened. Contents slimy and yeasty. Kidneys congested and pelves of, and ureters contain small blood clots. Urine bloody. Brain slightly congested. Blood and contents of bowels contained the same yeast vegetations as were found in the previous cases. Immediate cause of death, thrombosis and embolism.

CASE LXXV. Nov. 25. One hog only; died last night; weight 80 lbs.; poor. Had suffered severely with chronic diarrhœa for over three weeks. Trip-hammer pulsations began about eighteen hours before death. Surface blue. Lungs gorged with black, clotted blood, and contained many small tubercles, some of which are softening. Cavity of chest contained over one pint of bloody serum. Heart filled with blood clots and thrombi. Pericardium congested, with slight effusion of serum. Stomach and bowels congested and blackened, and contain in lower portions considerable jelly-like mucus and fermenting matter. Kidneys congested. Brain slightly congested. Blood and contents of bowels contained the same yeast vegetations found in the previous cases. Immediate cause of death, thrombosis and embolism.

CASE LXXVI. Nov. 26. Nine hogs have died since yesterday morning. The following are the post-mortems:—

(1.) Weight 160 lbs. Surface blue. Had chronic diarrhœa for over three weeks. Had trip-hammer pulsations for fourteen hours previous to death. Lungs gorged with black, clotted blood, and contained a few small tubercles. Cavity of chest contained about four ounces of effused serum. Heart filled with clots and thrombi. Liver gorged with black blood. Large intestines congested, thickened and filled with slimy mucus and fermenting food. Blood and contents of bowels contained same yeast vegetations as were present in all the previously examined cases. Immediate cause of death, thrombosis and embolism.

CASE LXXVII. (2.) Weight 165 lbs. Surface of body brightened. Had the appearance of capillary congestion over the whole cutaneous surface. Sick about four days. No trip-hammer pulsation of heart before death, such as is almost uniformly the case. Lungs quite healthy, but slightly congested. Heart apparently healthy, and blood very red and fluid. Liver on surface has a bluish tint. Kidneys and bladder healthy. Stomach congested; contents small, thin and yellow. Large intestines congested and thickened, and contained considerable jelly-like mucus. No tubercles in lungs. Brain congested. Blood and contents of bowels contain the same yeast vegetations as were found in the preceding cases. Cause of death, intense and persistent cutaneous congestion.

Case LXXVIII. (3.) Weight 120 lbs. In poor condition from having suffered with chronic diarrhœa, or consumption of the bowels, for three weeks. Trip-hammer pulsations began about fifteen hours before death. Surface blue. Lungs gorged with black, clotted blood, and contain many small tubercles. About half a pint of effused serum in cavity of chest. Heart congested and enlarged, and filled with blood clots and thrombi. Pericardium contained about two (2) ounces of effused serum. Liver gorged with black, clotted blood and softened. Kidneys gorged with blood and pelves of, contain blood clots. Stomach highly congested and contained sanguinous serum, mixed with mucus and fermenting food. Large intestines highly congested, thickened and partly filled with bloody serum, mucus and fermenting food. Brain slightly congested. Blood and contents of bowels contained the yeast vegetations mentioned in the previously examined cases. Immediate cause of death, thrombi and clots in heart, and emboli in lungs, liver, kidney and walls of stomach, and large intestines.

Case LXXIX. (4.) Weight 110 lbs. In poor condition from having suffered with severe chronic diarrhœa for about three weeks. Trip-hammer pulsations began about twelve hours before death. Surface natural. One lung gorged with black, clotted blood; the other only partially congested. Both lungs contained tubercles, some of which had broken down into creamy white matter like pus. About half a pint of effused serum in cavity of chest. Heart free from clots, but contained several small thrombi. Liver bluish and slightly softened. Stomach congested, thickened and contained a thin, lemon-colored slimy matter, mixed with fermenting food. Large intestines congested and thickened, and contents like that of the stomach. Brain congested, with slight effusion of serum. Blood contained the mycoderma aceti and the contents of the bowels the mycoderma aceti and the saccharomyces cerevisiæ. Immediate cause of death, thrombi in heart, and emboli in lungs and walls of stomach, and large intestines.

Case LXXX. (5.) Weight 130 lbs. In fair order. Had chronic diarrhœa for about ten days. Trip-hammer pulsations began sixteen hours before death. Surface blue. Lungs gorged with clotted blood and contained many small tubercles. Cavity of chest contained about one pint of effused serum. Pleura adherent to lungs in places. Heart contained blood clots and thrombi. Pericardium contained about three ounces of effused serum. Stomach dilated and filled with fermenting food. Large intestines thickened, congested and filled with fermenting food. Blood and contents of bowels contained the same yeast vegetations as were found in the previous case. Immediate cause of death, thrombi in heart and emboli in lungs.

Case LXXXI. (6.) Weight 140 lbs. In poor condition from having suffered with severe chronic diarrhœa for over three weeks. Trip - hammer pulsations began about twelve hours before death. Surface natural. One lung gorged with black, clotted blood; the other only partially congested. Walls of chest contained about one half pint of effused, bloody serum. One lung contained many small tubercles. Heart filled with blood clots and thrombi. Pericardium contained about two ounces of effused serum. Stomach congested, thickened and corrugated, and contained fermenting food, mixed with a slimy, yellow matter. Large intestines congested and thickened, and contained considerable jelly-like mucus mixed with fermenting food. Liver and kidneys gorged with black, clotted blood. Effused sanguinous serum in peritoneal cavity. Blood and contents of bowels contained the same yeast vegetations as previous cases. Immediate cause of death, thrombi in heart, and emboli in lungs, liver and kidneys.

Case LXXXII. (7.) Weight 90 lbs. Poor from having had chronic diarrhœa for three weeks. Surface natural. Trip-hammer pulsations began about fifteen hours before death. One lung gorged with black, clotted blood and the other only partially so ; contained many small tubercles. Cavity of chest contained about six ounces of effused serum. Pleura adherent in places. Heart filled with blood-clots and thrombi. Pericardium contained about one ounce of effused serum. Stomach and large intestines congested, thickened and contain mucus and fermenting food. Kidneys and liver blackened and gorged with clotted blood. Blood and contents of bowels contained the yeast vegetations found in previous cases. Immediate cause of death, thrombi in heart, and emboli in lungs, liver and kidneys.

Case LXXXIII. (8.) Weight 70 lbs. Quite poor from having suffered severely with consumption of bowels for fully three weeks. Trip-hammer pulsations began about twenty-four hours before death. Surface reddish all over. Liver congested and filled with red, clotted blood. Lungs partly gorged with red, clotted blood and contained many small tubercles. Cavity of chest contained about four ounces of effused serum. Heart filled with blood clots and small thrombi. Liver whitened and softened and undergoing fatty metamorphosis. Stomach and intestines congested and thickened, and contents fermenting and slimy. Blood contained the mycoderma aceti, and the contents of bowels, the mycoderma aceti and the saccharomyces cerevisiæ. Immediate cause of death, thrombi in heart and emboli in lungs with fatty liver.

Case LXXXIV. (9.) Weight 135 lbs. In good order. Has a large tubercular swelling on one ham that is partially broken down and ulcerating. Had chronic diarrhœa about ten days. Trip-hammer pulsations began about eighteen hours before death. Surface natural in color. One lung gorged with black, clotted blood and the other congested. Both lungs contained small tubercles. Cavity of chest contained one pint of effused serum. Heart contained small thrombi, but no blood clots. Pericardium contained about one ounce of effused serum.

Stomach congested and contents small, lemon-yellow and thin. Large intestines congested and thickened ; contents fermenting and slimy. Brain congested, with small effusion of serum. Blood and contents of bowels contained the same yeast vegetations as were found in previous cases. Immediate cause of death, thrombi in heart and emboli in lungs.

Case LXXXV. Nov. 27. Three hogs died since yesterday.

(1.) Weight 85 lbs. Poor from severe diarrhœa for three weeks. Trip-hammer pulsations began sixteen hours before death. Surface blue. Lungs gorged with black, clotted blood. Contained small tubercles breaking down. Heart filled with clotted blood and thrombi. Cavity of chest contained one pint of effused serum. Stomach and large intestines congested and thickened ; contents small, yellow, slimy and fermenting. Blood and contents of bowels contained the same kind of yeast vegetations previously found. Immediate cause of death, thrombi in heart and emboli in lungs.

Case LXXXVI. (2.) Weight 70 lbs. Poor from having suffered with chronic diarrhœa for over three weeks. Trip-hammer pulsations began fifteen hours before death. Surface natural color. Lungs only partially gorged with black, clotted blood. Cavity of chest contained about four ounces of effused serum. Lungs contained many small tubercles. Heart filled with clotted blood and thrombi. Pericardium contained about two ounces of effused serum. Stomach congested and filled with fermenting food. Large intestines thickened and filled with fermenting food and jelly-like mucus. Brain congested, with small effusion of serum. Blood and contents of bowels contained the same kind of yeast vegetations as were found in the previously described cases. Immediate cause of death, thrombi in heart and emboli in lungs.

CASE LXXXVII. (3.) Weight 80 lbs. Poor from having suffered with chronic diarrhœa for about three weeks. Triphammer pulsations began about seventeen hours before death. Surface blue. Lungs gorged with black, clotted blood and contained many small tubercles. Cavity of chest contained about one pint of effused, bloody serum. Pleura adherent in places. Heart filled with blood clots and thrombi. Stomach and large intestines congested, thickened and contained slimy mucus and fermenting food. Brain congested, with slight effusion. Blood and contents of bowels contained similar yeast vegetations to those previously examined. Immediate cause of death, thrombi in heart and emboli in lungs.

CASE LXXXVIII. Nov. 28. One hog died last night. Weight 100 lbs. Quite emaciated on account of having suffered with severe consumption of bowels for three weeks. Triphammer pulsations began about eighteen hours before death. Surface blue. Lungs gorged with black, clotted blood. Contained many small tubercles. Cavity of chest contained about one pint of effused serum. Pleura adherent to them in several places. Heart filled with blood clots and thrombi. Pericardium contained about three ounces of effused serum. Stomach highly congested and contained about one pint of lemon-yellow, slimy matter and fermenting food. Large intestines congested and thickened, and contained jelly-like matter and fermenting food. Liver gorged with black, clotted blood, and softened. Brain slightly congested. Other organs comparatively healthy. Blood contained numerous small groups of mycoderma aceti, and contents of bowels filled with the same vegetation, together with an abundance of alcoholic (saccharomyces cerevisiæ) yeast. Immediate cause of death, thrombi in heart and emboli in lungs and liver.

CASE LXXXIX. Nov. 29. One hog died last night in poor condition from having suffered severely, for over three weeks, with chronic diarrhœa. Trip-hammer pulsations began about eighteen hours before death. Surface blue. Lungs gorged with black, clotted blood, and contained many tubercles. Cavity of chest contained over one pint of effused bloody serum. Heart full of blood clots and white ropes of organized fibrin, extending through the heart and eight or ten inches down the aorta. Pericardium contained about four ounces of clear serum. Stomach and large intestines thickened and congested, and partially filled with slimy, yellow matter, mixed with fermenting food. Other organs comparatively healthy. Blood and contents of the bowels contained the same yeast vegetations as were found in the previously described cases. Immediate cause of death, thrombi in heart and emboli in lungs.

CASE XC. Nov. 30. Three hogs died last night.

(1.) Small sow; weight 80 lbs. In poor condition, from having suffered for over three weeks with severe chronic diarrhœa. Trip-hammer pulsations began about fourteen hours before death. Surface not blue. Lungs only partly filled with black, clotted blood; contained numerous small tubercles. Heart filled with blood clots and small thrombi. Pericardium contained about two ounces of effused serum. Stomach and large bowels congested and thickened, and contents contain slimy yellow matter mixed with fermenting food. Other organs healthy. Blood and contents of bowels contained the same kind of yeast vegetations as were found in the previously examined cases. Immediate cause of death, thrombi in heart and emboli in lungs.

CASE XCI. (2.) Sow heavy with pig. Weight 135 lbs. In fair order. Had chronic diarrhœa for about ten days. Trip-hammer pulsations began about ten hours before death. Surface not blue. Lungs only partially gorged with clotted blood. No tubercles could be found. Cavity of chest contained about two ounces of bloody serum. Heart contained a few clots and small thrombi. Pericardium contained about one ounce of effused serum. Stomach and large intestines congested, and the latter filled with a jelly-like matter mixed with fermenting food. Pigs dead and partially decayed. Kidneys and uterus highly congested and gorged with black, clotted blood. Blood and contents of bowels contained the same kind of yeast vegetations as were found in other previously examined cases. Immediate cause of death, thrombi in heart, and emboli in lungs, kidneys and uterine organs.

Case XCII. (3.) Weight 120 lbs. In poor condition, from having been sick with severe chronic diarrhœa for over three weeks. Trip-hammer pulsations began about twenty-four hours before death. Surface not blue. Lungs only partially gorged with black, clotted blood. Contained many small tubercles. Cavity of chest contained about six ounces of effused serum. Heart filled with blood clots and thrombi. Pericardium contained about four ounces of effused serum. Stomach congested and contained a small quantity of yellow, slimy matter, mixed with fermenting food. Large intestines highly congested and thickened, and filled with a jelly-like mucus and fermenting matter. Other organs comparatively healthy. Blood and contents of bowels contained the same kind of yeast vegetations as were found in the cases heretofore described. Immediate cause of death, thrombi in heart and emboli in lungs.

Case XCIII. Dec. 1. Three hogs died last night.
(1.) Weight 135 lbs. In fair order. Had chronic diarrhœa for about ten days. Trip-hammer pulsations began about ten hours before death. Surface blue. Lungs gorged with black, clotted blood; contained many small tubercles. Cavity of chest contained about one pint of effused serum. Heart filled with blood clots and thrombi. Pericardium contained about one ounce of effused serum. Liver gorged with black, clotted blood and softened. Stomach and intestines gorged with blood

and blackened, and contained fermenting food and mucus. Abdominal cavity contained about one pint of effused bloody serum. Brain congested with slight effusion of serum. Blood and contents of bowels full of the yeast vegetations found in previously described cases. Immediate cause of death, thrombi in heart and emboli in lungs, liver, stomach and intestines.

CASE XCIV. (2.) Weight 140 lbs. In fair condition. Suffered with chronic diarrhœa for over two weeks. Trip-hammer pulsations began about fourteen hours before death. Surface blue. Lungs gorged with black, clotted blood, and contained many small tubercles. Cavity of chest contained about one pint of effused bloody serum. Heart filled with blood clots and small thrombi. Pericardium contained about four ounces of effused serum. Liver gorged with clotted blood, and blackened and softened. Large intestines congested and thickened. Brain slightly congested. Other organs comparatively healthy. Blood and contents of bowels, full of the same kind of yeast vegetations discovered in the cases previously described. Immediate cause of death, thrombi in heart and emboli in lungs and liver.

CASE XCV. (3.) Weight 110 lbs. In rather poor condition from having suffered with chronic diarrhœa for about three weeks. Trip-hammer pulsations began about fourteen hours before death. Surface blue. Lungs gorged with black, clotted blood and contained small tubercles. Cavity of chest contained about four ounces of effused serum. Pleura contained about two ounces of serum. Heart filled with blood clots and thrombi. Stomach and large intestines congested, and partly filled with a jelly-like mucus and fermenting food. Brain slightly congested. Other organs comparatively healthy. Blood and contents of bowels contain the same kind of yeast vegetations found in the previously described cases. Immediate cause of death, thrombi in heart and emboli in lungs.

Case XCVI. Dec. 2. Four hogs died last night.

(1.) Barrow. Weight 115 lbs. Had chronic diarrhœa for over three weeks. Trip-hammer pulsations began about twelve hours before death. Surface natural. Lungs only partly gorged with black blood. Cavity of chest contained two or three ounces of serum. Could find no tubercles. Heart contained small thrombi but no clots. Intestines and stomach highly congested and blackened. Large intestines thickened and filled with a jelly-like mucus. Brain congested with small effusion of serum. Blood and contents of bowels contain the same yeast vegetations as were noticed in previous cases. Immediate cause of death, thrombi in heart and emboli in lungs, stomach and intestines.

Case XCVII. (2.) Weight 125 lbs. In fair condition. Had suffered with chronic diarrhœa for over three weeks. Trip-hammer pulsations began twelve hours before death, and were unusually severe. Surface blue. Lungs gorged with black, clotted blood, and cavity of chest contained one pint of bloody serum. Lungs contained many small tubercles. Heart filled with blood clots and thrombi. During the violent trip-hammer pulsations the heart was ruptured in region of right auricle. Large intestines congested and thickened, and filled with jelly-like mucus and fermenting food. Blood and contents of bowels contained the same kind of yeast vegetations found in the cases previously described. Immediate cause of death, thrombi in heart, rupture of heart, and emboli in lungs.

Case XCVIII. (3.) Weight 125 lbs. In fair order. Had chronic diarrhœa for about two and one half weeks. Trip-hammer pulsations began about fourteen hours before death. Surface natural in color. Lungs gorged with black, clotted blood, except the upper lobes; contained a few small tubercles. Cavity of chest contained about six ounces of effused serum. Heart filled with blood clots and thrombi. Pericardium contained about three ounces of effused serum. Stomach congested ; large intestines congested and thickened and partly filled with jelly-like mucus and fermenting food. Brain slightly congested. Other organs comparatively healthy. Blood contained masses of mycoderma aceti, and contents of bowels filled with vinegar (mycoderma aceti) and alcoholic (saccharomyces cerevisiæ) yeast. Immediate cause of death, thrombi in heart and emboli in lungs.

CASE XCIX. (4.) Weight 135 lbs. In fair order. Had chronic diarrhœa for about three weeks. Trip-hammer pulsations began about fifteen hours before death. Surface blue. Lungs gorged with black, clotted blood ; contained many small tubercles. Cavity of chest contained about eight ounces of effused serum. Pleura adherent in places. Heart filled with blood clots and thrombi. Pericardium contained about five ounces of effused serum. Liver white, fatty and softened. Stomach slightly congested. Large intestines congested and very much thickened, and contained a jelly-like mucus and fermenting food. Other organs comparatively healthy. Blood and contents of bowels contained the same kind of yeast vegetations as were found in the cases previously described. Immediate cause of death, thrombi in heart, emboli in lungs, and fatty liver.

CASE C. Dec. 3. Two hogs died last night. (1.) Weight 100 lbs. In poor condition, from having suffered with severe consumption of bowels (chronic diarrhœa) for over three weeks. Trip-hammer pulsations began about ten hours before death. Surface blue. Lungs gorged with black, clotted blood, and contained many small tubercles, some of which were softening. Cavity of chest contained about one pint of effused bloody serum. Pleura adherent in places. Heart filled with blood clots and small thrombi. Pericardium highly congested and contained about six ounces of effused serum. Stomach contained fermenting food and a lemon-yellow, slimy matter. Large intestines congested, very much thickened, and partly filled with jelly-like mucus and fermenting food. Kidneys congested and pelves of, contained small blood clots. Other organs comparatively healthy. Blood and contents of bowels contained the same kind of yeast vegetations found in previous cases.

CASE CI. (2.) Weight 95 lbs. In poor condition, from having suffered with severe chronic diarrhœa for about twenty days. Trip-hammer pulsations began about ten hours before death. Surface blue. Lungs gorged with black, clotted blood, and contained in upper portion small tubercles. Cavity of chest contained about six ounces of clear serum. Heart filled with blood clots and had several long thrombi passing through it and extending down in aorta. Pericardium contained about four ounces of effused serum. Liver gorged with black, clotted blood. Spleen highly congested. Stomach and large intestines highly congested and thickened, and contain slimy mucus and fermenting food. Kidneys congested, pelves and ureters contain small blood clots. Urine in bladder bloody. Other organs apparently healthy. Blood and contents of bowels contain the same kind of yeast vegetations as were found in the cases previously examined and described. Immediate cause of death, thrombi in heart and emboli in lungs, liver and kidneys.

CASE CII. Dec. 4. One hog died last night. Small. Weight 109 lbs. In rather poor condition, from having suffered about three weeks with chronic diarrhœa. Trip-hammer pulsations began about twelve hours before death. Surface blue. Lungs gorged with black, clotted blood, and contained many small tubercles. Cavity of chest contained about half a pint of effused bloody serum. Pleura adherent in several places. Heart filled with blood clots and had several small thrombi. Liver gorged with black blood and softened. Stomach and large intestines congested and thickened, and the latter filled with masses of jelly-like mucus and fermenting food. Cavity of abdomen contained about one pint of effused serum. Other organs comparatively healthy. Blood and contents of bowels contained the same kind of yeast vegetations found in the previous cases. Immediate cause of death, thrombi in heart and emboli in lungs and liver.

CASE CIII. Dec. 5. One hog died last night. Weight 130 lbs. In rather poor condition, from having suffered with chronic diarrhœa (consumption of the bowels) for about three weeks. Trip-hammer pulsations began about twelve hours before death. Surface blue. Lungs gorged with black, clotted blood, and contained several deposits of small tubercles, some of which were softening. Cavity of chest contained about one pint of bloody serum. Heart filled with blood clots, and several long thrombi of white organized fibrin, which extended some distance down into the aorta. Pleural cavity contains serum and deposits of lymph. Pericardium highly congested, and contained about six ounces of effused serum. Stomach congested. Large intestines congested and very much thickened, and partly filled with masses of jelly-like mucus and fermenting food. Other organs comparatively healthy. Blood and contents of the bowels contain the same kind of yeast vegetations found in the previously described cases. Immediate cause of death, thrombi in heart and emboli in lungs.

CASE CIV. Dec. 6. One hog died last night that had been sick with severe chronic diarrhœa for over three weeks. In rather poor flesh in consequence. Trip-hammer pulsations began about fourteen hours before death. Surface blue. Lungs gorged with black, clotted blood, and contained small tubercles in upper lobes. Pleura adherent in several places. Cavity of chest contained about one pint of effused bloody serum. Heart filled with blood clots and small thrombi. Pericardium contained about two ounces of effused serum. Liver gorged with black blood and softened. Diaphragm highly congested. Stomach and large intestines highly congested, and the latter very much thickened so as to greatly diminish the inside calibre of the organ. Kidneys highly congested and pelves of, and ureters filled with blood clots. Brain congested with small effusion of serum. Other organs comparatively healthy. Blood and contents of bowels contained the same kind of yeast vegetations as were found in cases previously described. Immediate cause of death, thrombi in heart and emboli in lungs, liver and kidneys.

With this CIVth case, end the records that were kept of post-mortem examinations. I made quite a number of others at other points, but did not keep records of them, as they corresponded so closely with those here given. I frequently visited the *pens* at the distilleries at and near Dresden and Zanesville, Muskingum County; those near Groveport; those near Dayton; those at Aurora, below Cincinnati; those at Richmond, above Cincinnati, and at various other points, to study the disease in these different localities, to detect differences — if any there might be — from varying situations, protections, exposures, hygienic conditions, weather, manner of feeding, and so on. In all cases I found the disease, in its genesis, natural history, pathological states and lesions, period of incubation and susceptibility, and that of immunity, the same. Wherever it prevailed to the greatest extent, then and there the slop was found to be more highly charged with acetic acid than at points where the percentages of deaths were less. Wherever the largest yield of whiskey — to the bushel of grain — was produced (other things being equal), there was the least acetic fermentation, the least acid in the slop, and the lowest death rate. In short, the death rate was found to vary with the varying amount of acetic acid in the slop. The greater the percentage of acetic acid in the food, the greater the death rate. While conducting the foregoing experiments, I took the precaution to feed hogs from the same localities, in adjoining pens, on good sound corn. The result was, that in no instance was there a trace of the disease, when the hogs were so fed. I did this, as there was a general impression, among distillers and pen-men, that the disease was to a greater or lesser extent infectious or contagious, and they were often careful to remove the hogs from the pens as soon as the "trip-hammer" pulsations began, regarding this last and fatal symptom in the malady as the specific disease itself. In all my observations and experience — for the past twenty years — in the feeding and fattening of hogs, I have never known a case of "Hog Cholera" among hogs fed on good, sweet, sound, unfermented and unfermenting food; and I doubt if such a case could occur, unless the hogs were closely confined, and so stuffed with highly diluted food that they could not digest at all. In this case, fermentative changes might be started in the digestive apparatus, which, if kept up for a sufficient length of time, might occasionally eventuate in the disease. Another factor enters into this problem, and that is a too large proportion of fluid taken with the solid food eaten. Other things being equal, the more the solid food is diluted with fluid (water) the greater is its liability to ferment. The reason of this is, that the water so dilutes the digestive fluids that they are too much weakened to dissolve the food. This is eminently a disease emanating from alcoholic and (especially) vinegar yeast, developed and developing, either already in the food eaten, or — under certain conditions — having its origin and subsequent development and accumulation in the digestive apparatus, after the same food is taken in. This latter state of things so rarely occurs that it would be of little moment. If the acid formed by the development of vinegar yeast is received into and developed in the system faster than it is eliminated, the whole organism, sooner or later, becomes so acid that the blood formed and forming becomes sticky and plastic, and by degrees shows a stronger tendency to thicken and to form thrombi and blood clots. Should this condition be established and sufficiently increase, a fatal thrombosis and embolism must result in course of time, as demonstrated by the preceding post-mortem chemical and microscopic examinations. All hogs fed upon this fermenting and highly acid food would soon perish, probably before the ninth or tenth week of the free feeding, were it not for one preventive, viz. : the natural tendency of the system to overcome obstacles and to gradually adapt itself to an abnormal diet. In such case the organism becomes able, little by little, to eliminate the morbid acid product as fast as it is taken in and formed.

The following résumé gives briefly the abnormal states and lesions in the 104 cases where post-mortems were made.

	No. of Cases.
Vinegar Yeast in Blood	104
Vinegar and Alcoholic Yeast in Digestive Organs	104
Consumption of Bowels, or Chronic Diarrhœa	104
Embolism	104
Thrombosis — producing " trip-hammer " pulsations	103
Embolism in Lungs	102
Thrombi and blood clots found in Heart after death	88
Thrombi and blood clots dislodged from Heart before death	15
Embolism in Kidneys	55
Embolism in Liver	43
Embolism in Genital Organs	7
Embolism in Stomach and Intestines	75
Embolism in Diaphragm	11
Embolism in Omentum	2
Embolism in Mesentery	4
Embolism in Muscles of Abdomen	1
Cutaneous Embolism	2
Embolism in Spleen	5
Embolism in Brain, resulting in effusion	72
Effusion in Pericardium	37
Effusion in Chest	85
Effusion in Abdominal cavity	9
Thickening of large Intestines	82
Tubercles in Lungs	79
Tubercles in Intestinal walls and Lungs	6

Tubercles in Intestinal walls and not in Lungs . . .		12
Tubercles in Mesentery		1
Surface of body blue before and after death		56
Heart ruptured during "trip-hammer" pulsations . . .		1
Abscess in Kidneys		1
Ruptured blood-vessels in Lung		45
Ruptured blood-vessels in Kidneys		35
Ruptured blood-vessels in Ureters		12
Ruptured blood-vessels in Liver		6
Ruptured blood-vessels in Intestinal walls		5
Ruptured blood-vessels in Brain		16
Ruptured blood-vessels in Pericardium		8
Ruptured blood-vessels in Mesentery		4
Ruptured blood-vessels in female Genital Organs . . .		6
Ruptured blood-vessels in Peritoneum		3

The effusion in and around the various organs blocked up with emboli seems to have been greatly caused by the obstructed blood-vessels in the parts, together with the severe pressure produced by the violent spasmodic beating of the heart for the few hours previous to death. In many cases, this pressure was so great as to cause a rupture of the blood-vessels.

It will be seen from the foregoing summary that vinegar yeast (mycoderma aceti) was found in the blood of all 104 cases examined. The acid yeast occurred in small, usually elongated groups of spores, distributed quite abundantly throughout the blood, as seen in Plate XVIII.

Figs. 1 and 2, Pl. XVIII, are fair representations of " Hog Cholera" blood. One of these drawings, Fig. 1, was made from a sample of the blood of Case 8. The upper portions of the lungs contained many small tubercles. Fig. 2 was made from the blood of Case 79. Small tubercles were found in all parts of the lungs, some of them having broken down. The fibrin filaments in the blood are much contracted in length, which increases their diameter and visibility, and at the same time lessens the size of the meshes through which, in health, the blood discs freely flow. This diminution of the meshes obstructs the free passage of blood discs, in consequence of which the blood aggregates in strings, masses and ropes, becoming partially clotted. The blood discs and colorless corpuscles also become sticky and plastic. Such blood, when placed between the slides of the microscope, instead of spreading out evenly and covering all the field alike, becomes aggregated in strings, irregular rows and masses, leaving vacant spaces, wherein are seen only the fibrin filaments, and here and there the elongated masses of the spores of the mycoderma aceti, or vinegar yeast.

Vinegar yeast (mycoderma aceti), Fig. 3, Pl. XIX, and alcoholic yeast (saccharomyces cerevisiæ), Fig. 4, Pl. XIX, were found abundantly in the fermenting contents of the bowels in all of the 104 cases. These were also as abundantly found in all the yeasty diarrhœal passages before death. The constant fermentation and development of these vegetations in the large bowels gave rise to the secretion, largely, of a jelly-like mucus, which kept the mucus follicles constantly blocked up and congested. This congestion continued, and resulted in the thickening of the internal walls of the colon and rectum. In some cases, the large bowels had become so filled up by this thickening, that the passage was almost entirely closed. Consumption of the bowels, or chronic diarrhœa (Hog Cholera), occurred in all the 104 cases, and lasted from one to four or five weeks, before the fatal attack of thrombosis and embolism. These were always indicated by the "trip-hammer" pulsations in heart, which were so violent that in one case the heart was ruptured, and in many cases, blood-vessels were burst in the organs that were filled with the emboli. In still many more cases there were extensive effusions in the obstructed organs. Embolism occurred in all the 104 cases; although a simple side issue in the disease, it was in every instance the immediate cause of death. Thrombosis, which with the embolism caused the "trip-hammer" pulsations, was present in 103 of the 104 cases. The single instance where there were no "trip-hammer" pulsations was Case 77, where there was a bright scarlet redness

over the whole surface, and extreme cutaneous congestion or
embolism.   There was embolism in the lungs in 102 of the 104
cases.   The two cases where there was no embolism were the
two cases of cutaneous embolism.   Thrombi and blood clots
were found in the heart after death in 88 of the 104 cases.
In the balance of the cases, fifteen in number, of thrombosis
producing "trip-hammer" pulsations, the thrombi and blood
clots had been dislodged from the heart previous to death.
There was embolism in the kidneys in 55 of the 104 cases,
and in several of these the blood-vessels of the kidneys were
ruptured from the force with which the blood was pressed into
them by the violent heart pulsations.   In 43 of the 104 cases,
there was embolism in the liver, with rupture of the blood-vessels in the organ, in several of them.   There was embolism in
the female genital organs in seven cases, in six of which blood-
vessels were ruptured.   There was embolism in the stomach
and intestines in 75 cases.   Embolism in omentum in two
cases.   Embolism in abdominal muscles, with extreme rupture
of blood-vessels in the parts, in one case.   Cutaneous embolism
in two cases ; one of these was the only instance, in the 104
cases, where there were no "trip-hammer" pulsations of heart
before death.   Embolism in spleen in five cases.   Embolism in
brain, resulting in more or less effusion, in 72 cases.   There
was effusion in pericardium in 37 cases.   Effusion in cavity of
chest in 85 cases.   Effusion in abdominal cavity in nine cases.
There was thickening in the walls of large intestines in 82
cases, in some of which the passage had become almost oc-
cluded.   Tubercles were found in the lungs in 79 of the 104
cases.   They were small and recently formed.   Tubercles were
found both in the intestinal walls and lungs in six cases.   Tubercles were found in intestinal walls and not in lungs in 12 cases.
The surface of the body was blue both before and after death
in 56 cases.   The heart was found ruptured, by the severe
"trip-hammer" pulsations, in one case only.   The blood-vessels of the lungs were ruptured in 45 cases.   The blood-vessels

of the kidneys were ruptured in 35 cases. The blood-vessels of the ureters were ruptured in 12 cases. The blood-vessels of the liver were ruptured in 6 cases. The blood-vessels of the intestines were ruptured in 5 cases. The blood-vessels of the brain were ruptured in 16 cases. The blood-vessels of the pericardium were ruptured in 8 cases. The blood-vessels of the mesentery were ruptured in 4 cases. The blood-vessels of the female genital organs were ruptured in 6 cases. The blood-vessels in peritoneum were ruptured in 3 cases. Abscess of the kidneys in one case. Gall-bladder and gall ducts were clogged with intestinal worms in one case. Intestines were partially blocked up with tape-worms in one case. The main cause of the extensive and numerous effusions, and the frequent rupture of blood-vessels, is, no doubt, the great pressure produced upon the blocked-up blood-vessels, by the violent "trip-hammer" pulsations of the heart during the last few hours of life. The mucous secretions in the fauces and lungs were thick, sticky and ropy, and contained vinegar yeast (mycoderma aceti), Fig. 5, Pl. XIX, and alcoholic yeast (saccharomyces cerevisiæ), Fig. 6, Pl. XIX. The vinegar yeast was much more abundant in them than the alcoholic.

Fig. 7, Pl. XIX, represents capillary embolism : *a* represents a small artery; *b*, a branch of same; and *c, c, c, c*, branchlets, which, after subdividing still further, finally terminate in capillary vessels, *e, e, e, e.* The terminal arteries and their outgoing capillary vessels are all filled or plugged up with emboli. Fig. 8, Pl. XIX, represents an arterial extremity (*f*) with its outgoing capillary vessels, *g, g, g*, highly magnified, all blocked up with emboli or blood clots. These two illustrations display the condition of the blood-vessels in Hog Cholera, in all the organs affected with embolism. These emboli are pushed along in the blood stream as far as they can be forced by the powerful "trip-hammer" pulsations of the heart, till finally the minuteness of the blood-vessels precludes their further advance.

Then there is a sudden standstill, a damming up of the stream; frequently this reacts with such force as to rupture blood-vessels.

Prevention and Treatment.

Hog Cholera is strictly and preëminently a disease of abnormal and unhealthy alimentation. It is produced by food undergoing a process of metamorphosis which develops in it substances that can neither be appropriated to the support of the tissues, nor yet be eliminated with a readiness sufficient to prevent their producing grave disturbances in the state of the blood, and in the condition of vital organs. These products are developed in the food by alcoholic and acetic fermentations, and are alcohol, acetic acid, and alcoholic and acid yeasts. The acetic acid, being taken in faster than it can be eliminated, accumulates little by little, rendering the system more and more acid, till finally the organism is so saturated with it that the blood in process of formation in the mesenteric glands and spleen, gradually becomes sticky, stringy and viscous, and takes on the formation of clots. This continues step by step, till blood clots and thrombi are actually formed, and when these break loose and go floating along the blood stream, fatal embolism may result.

The injurious effects of the acetic acid are increased by the gradual absorption of carbonic acid gas, with which the stomach and bowels are constantly filled. This gas slowly paralyzes the muscles, follicles and glands of the whole digestive apparatus, so that these surfaces, villi and follicles cease to have the selective power of health, through which to carry on the various normal physiological processes : deleterious products then effect an entrance together with the nutritious. This state being ushered in, diaphragm, heart, lungs, the whole organism in fact, begin to get more and more enervated. The action of the heart weakens ; the extremities are colder ; the breathing is more hurried and labored ; the nerves of sense are more or less paralyzed : all of which aggravates the effects of the acetic acid by partially paralyzing the entire system and preventing such a rapid elimination of the acetic acid as might otherwise take place. The yeast is still another factor in the problem, besides the part it plays in metamorphosing healthy food into disease-producing materials. The vinegar yeast (mycoderma aceti) in the blood forms little emboli which may block up the minute capillary vessels in the lungs ; the intestinal walls ; the mesenteric, lymphatic and other glands, and those of other organs : nuclei for the little deposits known as tubercles are thus formed. The vinegar and alcoholic yeasts may also form masses and plugs in the mucous follicles of the lungs and digestive apparatus, which masses and plugs may become too large to be discharged : in this case they likewise form nuclei for another class of deposits, which are extra-vascular, and which also become tubercles. Hence it will be seen that the yeast is the primary as well as the secondary cause of those dreaded diseases, consumption of the bowels (Hog Cholera), and consumption of the lungs, or tubercular phthisis. This whole matter is fully and clearly set forth in another part of this work.

Now, if the fermenting, sour food is the cause of " Hog Cholera," — of which fact there is no shadow of doubt, — the disease is easily cured if taken before the trip-hammer pulsations begin ; also one which is readily prevented by avoiding that kind of food which produces it.

After the trip-hammer pulsations have set in, the lesions and pathological states are too great to admit of a cure. In ninety-nine cases out of a hundred, the hog is then past all help. But any time previous to this the cure is simple and easy. Stop all fermenting and acid food. Feed sound corn, or any other sweet, normal " hog food." Keep the hog quiet, avoiding all active and severe exercise. The blood will gradually lose its sticky, plastic, tough condition, the diarrhœa will cease, and in a few weeks the hog is well and hearty. If it be desirable to continue the feeding of the sour, fermenting slop, much can be done in the way of lessening the death-rate, by neutralizing the food with lime and chalk before feeding. To treat the disease medicinally, while continuing the cause (acid, fermenting food), is a labor by no means attended with uniform success. Much can be done, however, by neutralizing the slop with lime, chalk and soda, when it is hot and fresh from the stills, stirring it well and frequently. It should then be allowed to stand and settle for several hours : just before feeding, add a little sulphur and salt. Anything warming, like pepper or ginger, added to the food, aids the digestive process.

This, however, does not prevent the disease. It only lessens the death-rate and enables you to get more diseased hogs fat enough for the slaughter-house. Every hog fattened upon sour, fermenting food is a consumptive hog, and if allowed to continue long enough on this diet, would sooner or later die of this disease.

Although the hogs undoubtedly have consumption, and though the meat is meat of unsound and diseased animals, yet I hardly think it is ever the real cause of consumption in man, although when freely eaten it may aggravate the fermentation of farinaceous and saccharine food, and in this way become a collateral aid in developing the true cause of the disease in man.

As it would be a great loss to the distiller to throw away the " slop " of his establishment, while on the other hand it is dangerous to feed hogs exclusively upon it before their system becomes able to digest, assimilate and eliminate it without ill effects, it becomes important to know to what extent, in an economical point of view, it may be safely used. In repeated experiments in this direction, it has been found that hogs may gradually become used to this kind of food, so that, after a certain period, they may be able to digest, assimilate and eliminate the good and bad products of the " slop," till they become sufficiently fat to slaughter, without any very serious results as regards death-rate. This is brought about by beginning to feed the " slop " in small quantities at first, the balance of the food being good sound corn ; gradually increasing the slop and decreasing the corn from week to week till about the end of the eighth week of feeding. The corn is then so reduced in proportion to the " slop " that it can be safely left out. From this time on, the hogs seem to be able to digest and assimilate the " slop," and eliminate the acetic acid so as to prevent dangerous derangements. Begin by feeding for the first seven days but one gallon of "slop " per day to each hog, the balance of feed being good sound corn. From the seventh to the fourteenth day, feed two gallons of " slop " per day to each hog. From the fourteenth to the twenty-first day, feed three gallons of " slop " per day to each hog. From the twenty-first to the twenty-eighth day, feed four gallons of slop per day to each hog, and so on, increasing the amount of slop to each hog every seventh day one gallon, till, at the end of the eighth week, each hog gets eight gallons per day, which is about the amount required per hog for full feed. During the gradual increase in the " slop " to each hog, the sound corn fed is lessened weekly as the " slop " is increased, till finally, at the beginning of the ninth week, the corn is left off entirely. In this way the hogs gradually become used to the acid " slop," so that they are able to eliminate the acetic acid with sufficient rapidity to prevent any very serious results.

If care be taken to carry out this mode of feeding with exactitude, the death-rate will be comparatively light. The hogs, however, are all consumptive animals, but the disease does not advance with sufficient rapidity, to prevent them from fattening quickly, and if not kept too long on this diet, they may pass for comparatively healthy hogs. If sufficient care be taken in feeding, the hogs — for the most part — escape death from thrombus and embolism, which otherwise would occur mostly from the third to the end of the eighth week. Hogs should never be turned into a field of corn and allowed to harvest it themselves. The corn should be husked and fed to the hogs on clean, dry floors, and only fed daily in quantities that will be cleanly eaten up. In this way the corn is always sound and sweet, and none is allowed to ferment and sour before being eaten. Hog cholera, like consumption in man, is transmissible by inoculation. All diseases that arise from the development of vegetable or animal organisms, on or in the tissues, are or may be communicated by inoculation. It is like inoculating a piece of dough with yeast, or any organic matter with its ferment. The smallest amount of matter from a cadaver in a certain stage of decomposition (or fermentation) excites a like condition in the living body when inoculated in it.

From these experiments we learn this important lesson : *even hogs cannot " make hogs of themselves " with impunity, on a diet that their digestive organs were never made to properly digest and assimilate.* The structure and functions of the digestive apparatus in each class of the animal kingdom, determine its natural and healthy food. Upon this alone can it live without producing disease ; upon this it thrives, and if discreetly fed, it escapes all those fatal chronic maladies which arise from long-continued abnormal alimentation.

This fact is so vital, not alone to animals, but also, and in even greater degree, to MAN, that I may be pardoned if I repeat, in closing my work — *Nearly all the diseases that "flesh is heir to," aside from those produced by parasites, poisons and injuries in general, are the terrible outcome of defective and unhealthy feeding.*

With the mass of evidence herein presented, I may safely rest my case for the time being, content with having called thoughtful attention to a great but much ignored TRUTH. It is my abiding hope that the PEOPLE may be brought to see these facts for themselves, and may by individual and intelligent self-control aid their physicians to restore and maintain the oft-imperiled balance of HEALTH. Without it there is neither BEAUTY, USE, nor HAPPINESS for us : in its absence all the great glories and truths fade away from our sick vision. If we will not learn from NATURE's methods, she crushes us in the reversion of her laws, and passes on. But if we examine and inaugurate her processes, we become as calm and as strong as she, and, like her, in our lives we receive and manifest the DIVINE.

LVII.

DIET IN PREGNANCY AND DURING THE NURSING PERIOD. THE
NATURAL FOOD FOR INFANTS.

IF women would live healthfully, that is, upon such foods
as they can well digest and assimilate, and would keep their
stomachs clean, the urine clear and standing at a density of
about 1.015, and the bowels moving regularly once a day,
there would then always be healthy downward peristalsis in the
muscles and nerves of organic life. The system would be free
from sufferings and aches, the pains of childbirth would be few
and easily borne, and the labors short, lasting only from a few
minutes to two hours. Under the above states and conditions
there is natural downward peristaltic action in the womb. As
LABOR sets in, the muscles of the uterus begin to contract at the
fundus and move downwards towards the neck, while those of
the neck and os relax and open to the pressure from above.
Sometimes the child is expelled by a single pain; at others, it
requires from two to half a dozen expulsive efforts, and at still
others, from six to a dozen.

Healthy Alimentation.

The alimentation productive of health is about two parts of
lean meat food to one of vegetable food. The best lean meats
are beef and mutton. Chicken, fish, eggs and game, may be
brought in as side dishes. Oysters may be taken either raw,
plain broiled, or roasted in the shell.

The best vegetable foods are bread, toast, cracked wheat,
boiled rice, hominy, potatoes, green peas (fresh from vines) and
string beans freshly picked. The rice and cracked wheat should

be boiled about three hours in a double vessel with a water jacket, and the hominy boiled in the same kind of vessel at least six hours. This changes the starch into glucose, which is one step in the digestive process.

The vegetable foods should not be used to the extent of producing flatulence. Fruits should be sparingly eaten, and only after one meal in the day. Tomatoes and celery may be moderately used as relishes.

About one pint of hot water should be drank an hour and a half before each meal and on retiring. The purpose of this water-drinking is to cleanse out the stomach for the meals and for the rest at night.

It is desirable to rest at least half an hour before and after eating, and during this rest to be passive and free from care, anxiety and any mental effort. No matter what troubles exist, it is possible and necessary to banish them by self-control at this time. Tired nature will rest, if only we permit it, by abandoning ourselves to passivity and relaxation. The meals should not be tasks, but enjoyable recreations, with ease, smiles and laughter as valuable condiments. If we seek, we can always find cause for contentment and a smile.

After childbirth, the mother should continue her substantial and healthy diet through the period of lactation. Her milk will then be of the best, and will nourish and build up the child most happily, relieving it from the tortures, screams and great fatalities of babyhood : it will then be a model of loveliness, sweetness and pleasure to its parents and to all concerned.

Food, and Mode of Feeding the Child.

As soon as born, the baby should be washed in warm water, wrapped in a soft blanket and put to the breast. This first milk is what the child requires.

From this time until the appearance of the front teeth, no food but the mother's milk should be given to the child. The baby should be nursed about every three hours with regularity, and given but little at a time; no more than it can well digest without fermentation. The quietude of the baby, and its freedom from flatulence and colic pains, will be a guide to the mother in this respect. After nursing comes quiet and rest. Infants should eat, sleep and be happy. This should be their only occupation.

When the meat or front teeth begin to show themselves, NATURE tells us that the time has arrived when a little meat food would be desirable. It should be brought in, in the way of beef juice and beef pulp. This should at first be given simply as a side dish and in small quantity. As more meat teeth appear, more meat may be given, the diet consisting of lean meat and milk only.

When the vegetable, or double teeth begin to make their appearance, NATURE suggests that the period has come to bring in a little bread and vegetable food, but only as adjuncts to the previous milk and meat diet.

The proportion should be small at first, but can be gradually increased, care being observed not to give these fermentable aliments in sufficient quantity to cause fermentation and flatulence.

When the mother is unable to nurse her child for want of milk, a wet-nurse, or cow's milk (fresh), should be substituted. The various manufactured baby foods should be given a wide berth, if it is in any way possible to avoid them. Weaning from the mother's milk should take place when the child is from twelve to eighteen months old, or earlier if from any cause the mother's milk should become poor in nutritious elements.

The simple plans here briefly set forth are the outcome of our natural structure. Nature gives us these plain indications in our make-up. As fully stated elsewhere in these pages, we have twenty meat teeth and only twelve vegetable teeth. The stomach (the first and largest organ of the digestive apparatus) digests nothing but lean meats, while the small bowels, with the secretions of the liver, pancreas and glands of Lieberkuhn and Brunner, digest vegetable foods and fat.

We are thus about two thirds carnivorous and one third herbivorous, and if we live according to this structure — other conditions being favorable — there need be but little danger of our ever getting out of order.

The great accomplishment in life is to be able to read and understand as correctly as possible the meaning of everything that comes in the range of our experience. It is well known that all objects and living beings in nature, and the individual elements, parts and organs of which they are composed, are each and every one symbols of ideas. They together make up a natural language, by which the universal mind expresses itself truthfully and in a way so simple and plain that the student of Nature cannot fail to understand the full and complete meaning.

LVIII.

DOWNWARD AND UPWARD PERISTALSIS.

In the healthy state of man in his normal condition, all physical actions travel from the head to the feet, and all psychic actions from the feet to the head. These actions may be called downward peristalsis and upward peristalsis. Downward peristalsis travels with considerable regularity the entire length of the body about every minute. When these actions go on continuously, one wave succeeding the other with regularity, we feel well, and all goes on happily. This vital influence travels in the sympathetic nerves or nerves of organic life, and through them manifests itself in the organic muscular fibres of the vascular system, glandular system and digestive apparatus. Through the nerve extremities it reaches also every part of the epithelial and endothelial surfaces and their glandular appendages.

Reverse the downward action in the nervous system, and there is a tendency to epilepsy: in the digestive apparatus, and there is biliousness, headaches, congestions and fullness about the head, and often a tendency to nausea and vomiting. In any of the eruptive fevers this reversed action may so aggravate the disease as to cause death.

These downward and upward actions are greatly under our own control. To influence them we must be perfectly passive, retiring back in ourselves, endeavoring to live all over alike, peacefully and contentedly. If our thoughts are running wild, flying off in every direction without aim or purpose, we should calmly and quietly withdraw the thoughts from the outer world and direct our attention to the quiet expanse within the entire body, fix ourselves there, and then listen and wait.

If we are calmly persistent in this soul effort, a pleasant thrill will soon begin to pervade the body ; strength and repose will creep over and through us, normal upward and downward actions will assume control, and a feeling of comfort, satisfaction and peace with all the world will take possession of us. So long as we yield ourselves up in this way to nature and " possess our souls in patience," we are gradually growing better and better. As we gain, this internal attitude need not be confined to moments of rest and quiet alone, but may pervade active life and loosen its strain and fever.

EXPLANATION OF THE PLATES.

PLATE I. *Figs.* 1, 2 and 3. Casts containing crystals from the follicles of the large bowels, in Chronic Diarrhœa.

Figs. 4 to 34. Various vegetations found developing in the mucous secretions of the large bowels in Chronic Diarrhœa.

PLATE II. *Figs.* 10 to 41. The various vegetations found in the mucous passages of consumption of the bowels. Also appearance of crystalline fat (seroline) in passages.

PLATE III. *Figs.* 1, 2, 3 and 4. Appearance and state of fibrin filaments in blood in health and in different diseases.

PLATE IV. *Fig.* 1. Appearance of blood in man at maturity, where there is perfect health and a good constitution.

Fig. 2. Appearance of blood in infancy, where there is perfect health and a good constitution.

PLATE V. *Fig.* 1. Appearance of blood in Eczema, with the vegetation that causes the disease.

Fig. 2. Appearance of blood in the later stages of Anæmia.

PLATE VI. *Fig.* 1. Appearance of blood with skeins of fibrin filaments in it, in Fibræmia.

Fig. 2. Skeins of fibrin filaments as seen in the blood in Fibræmia.

PLATE VII. Skeins of fibrin floating in the blood stream as emboli, in Fibræmia.

PLATE VIII. *Fig.* 1. Appearance of blood in the last part of the first stage, and early part of second stage of Tubercular Consumption.

Fig. 2. Appearance of the blood in the last part of the second stage of Tubercular Consumption.

PLATE IX. *Figs.* 1 and 2. Appearance and condition of blood in last part of the third stage of Consumption.

PLATE X. Appearance and condition of blood in the early part of the fourth stage of Tubercular Consumption.

PLATE XI. *Figs.* 1 and 2. Appearance of blood in the last part of the fourth stage of Tubercular Consumption.

PLATE XII. Represents blood of patients in the last stage of Tubercular

Consumption, when they have been on the diet treatment for (*Fig.* 1) three months, and for (*Fig.* 2) six months, showing the changes that have taken place in the direction of improvement and cure.

PLATE XIII. *Fig.* 1. Blood in Fibrous Consumption.

Fig. 2. Rheumatic Blood.

PLATE XIV. *Figs.* 1 to 16. Spores of acid yeasts in the expectoration of Consumption. *Figs.* 17 to 23. Spores of a yeast vegetation developing in the skin, in Tubercular Consumption.

Figs. 43, 46 and 49. Spores and filaments of leptothrix, found in the sputa of Consumption.

Figs. 50 to 55. Vegetations found in the sputa of Tubercular Consumption.

Fig. 78. Shreds of breaking-down connective tissue, found in the sputa of the last stage of Consumption.

PLATE XV. *Figs.* 24, 66, 67, 68 and 76. Spores of a yeast vegetation developing in the skin, in the later stages of Tubercular Consumption.

Figs. 25 to 40, 42, 56, 57, 61, 62, 63, 64, 70, 71, 72, 73, 74, 75 and 77. Vegetations in the expectoration, in the last or breaking-down stage of Tubercular Consumption.

PLATE XVI. *Figs.* 1 to 4. Various appearances of cells of ciliated epithelium as expectorated in Asthma.

Figs. 5, 6, 7, 10, 12, 13, 17, 18, 19, 25, 26, 31, 32 and 54. Various appearances of the giant cells expectorated in Asthma.

Figs. 14, 20, 21, 22, 23, 24, 27, 28, 29, 34 to 38. Crystals and calculi found in expectorations of Asthma.

Figs. 49, 50, 51, 55, 56, 58 and 62. Appearances of some of the vegetations developing in the sputa of Asthma.

Figs. 8, 9 and 11. Albuminoid matter (undergoing amœboid changes) escaped from the giant cells.

PLATE XVII. *Figs.* 39, 40, 41 and 42. Calculi coughed up in gravel of the lungs, or Asthma.

Figs. 44 to 47. Double fusiform crystals in asthmatic expectoration.

Fig. 48. Spore of species of fucidium.

Figs. 63, 66, 71, 72, 73, 74, 82 to 88. Various vegetations found in sputa of Asthma.

Figs. 76 to 80. Species of spirulina developing in the air cells in Asthma.

PLATE XVIII. *Figs.* 1 and 2. Appearance and condition of blood in swine, when they have died of Tubercular Consumption and Consumption of Bowels.

PLATE XIX. *Figs.* 3 to 6. Alcoholic and acid yeast plants in Consumption of Bowels in Hogs.

Figs. 7 and 8. Arterial extremities blocked with Emboli; Thrombosis and Embolism in hogs.

PLATE I.

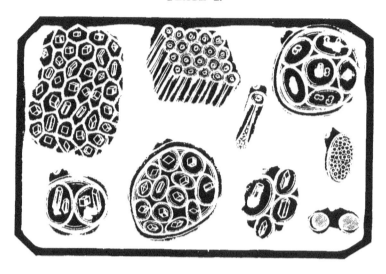

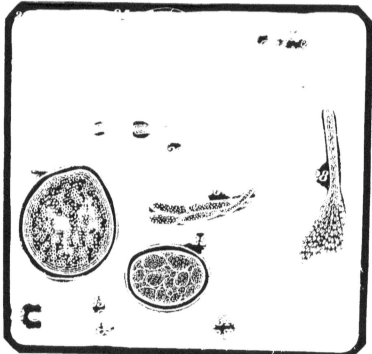

Figs. 1, 2, and 3. — Casts containing crystals from the follicles of the large bowels in chronic diarrhœa.

Figs. 4–34. — Various vegetations found developing in the mucous secretions of the larger bowels in chronic diarrhœa.

PLATE II.

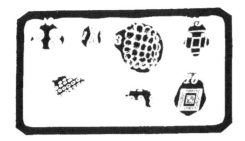

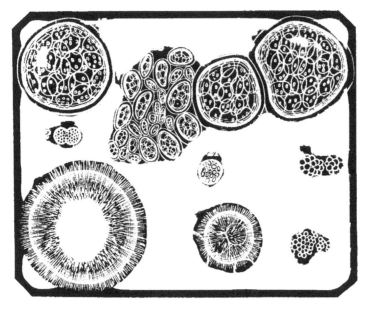

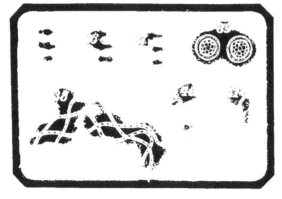

Figs. 10–41. — The various vegetations found in the mucous passages of consumption of the bowels.   Also appearance of crystalline fat (seroline) in passages.

PLATE III.

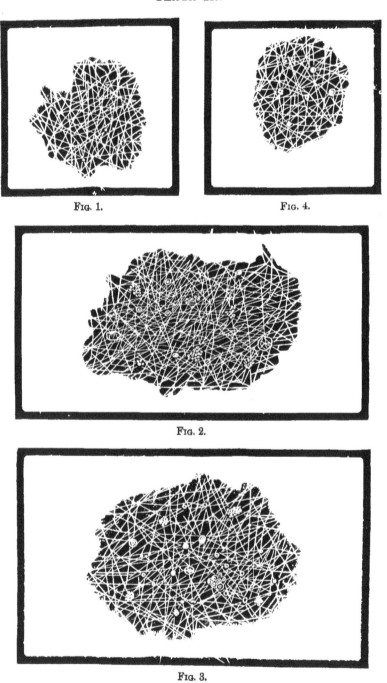

Fig. 1.   Fig. 4.

Fig. 2.

Fig. 3.

Fig. 1.   Appearance and state of fibrin filaments in blood in health ; 2, 3, 4, in different diseases.

PLATE IV.

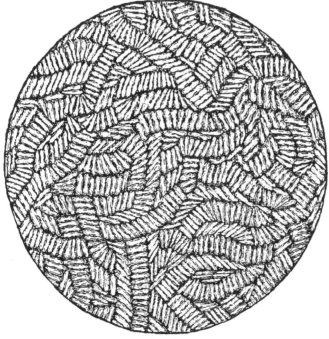

FIG. 1.

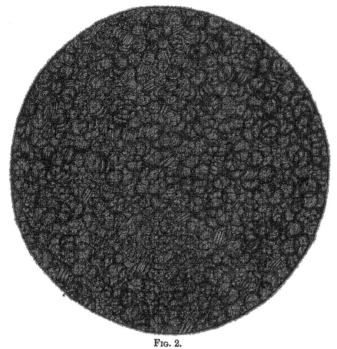

FIG. 2.

Fig. 1. — Healthy blood in adult of good constitution.
Fig. 2. — Healthy blood in infant of good constitution.

PLATE V.

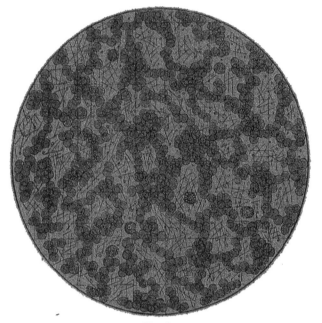

Fig. 1.

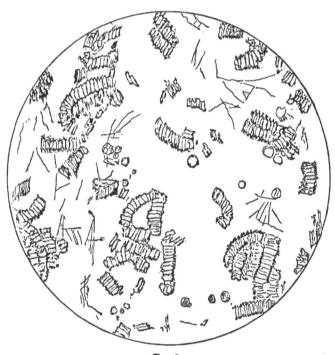

Fig. 2.

Fig. 1.—Appearance of blood in eczema, with the vegetation that causes the disease.
Fig. 2.—Appearance of blood in the later stages of anæmia.

PLATE VI.

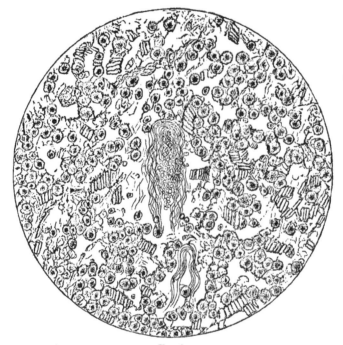

Fig. 1.

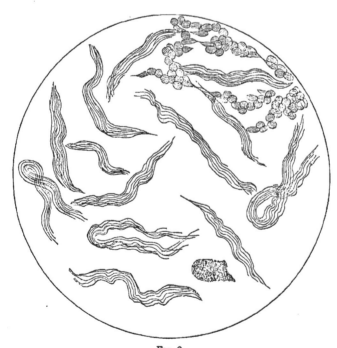

Fig. 2.

Fibræmia.

PLATE VII.

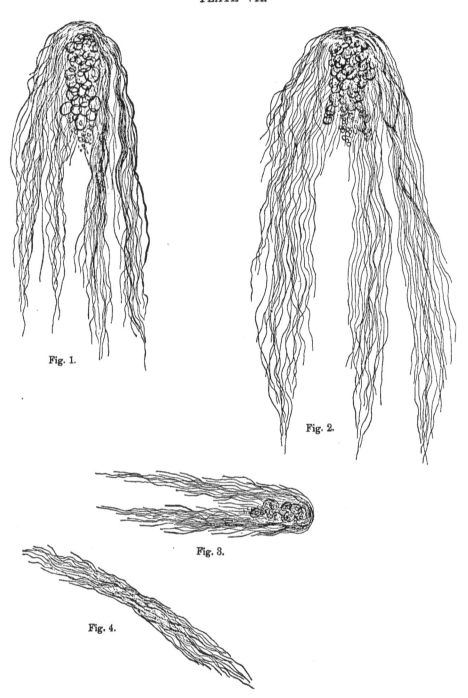

Fig. 1.

Fig. 2.

Fig. 3.

Fig. 4.

Skims of fibrin floating in the blood stream as emboli, in fibræmia.

PLATE VIII.

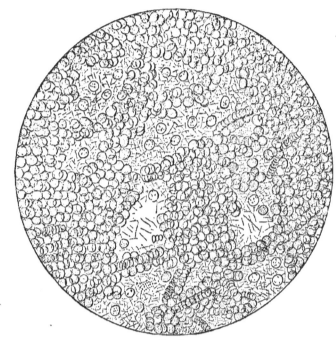

Fig. 1.

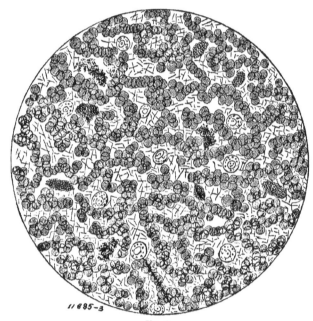

Fig. 2.

Fig. 1.— Appearance of blood in the last part of the first and early part of the second stage of tubercular consumption.

Fig. 2. — Appearance of blood in the last part of the second stage of tubercular consumption.

PLATE IX.

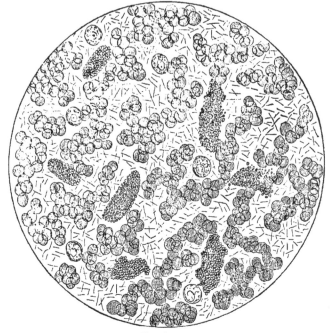

FIG. 1.

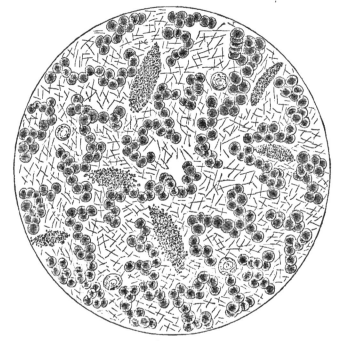

FIG. 2.

Figs. 1 and 2. — Appearance and condition of blood in last part of the third stage of consumption.

PLATE X.

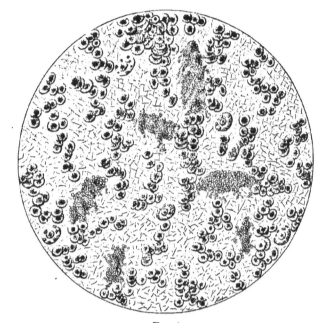

FIG. 1.

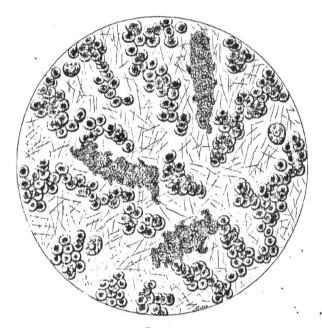

FIG. 2.

Figs. 1 and 2.—Appearance and condition of blood in the early part of the fourth stage of tubercular consumption.

PLATE XI.

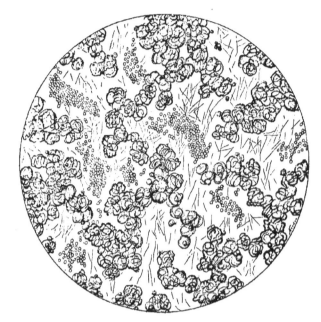

FIG. 1.

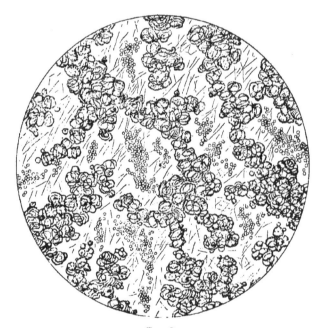

FIG. 2.

Figs. 1 and 2.—Appearance of blood in the last part of the fourth stage of tu er-
cular consumption.

PLATE XII.

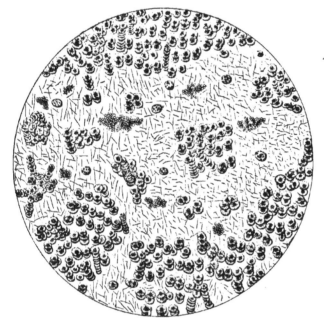

FIG. 1.

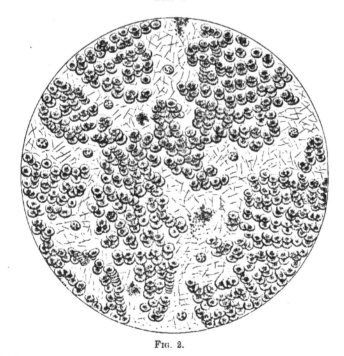

FIG. 2.

Fig. 1.—Appearance and condition of blood in fourth stage of tubercular phthisis, after six months' treatment.

Fig. 2.—Appearance and condition of blood in fourth stage of tubercular phthisis, after twelve months' treatment.

PLATE XIII.

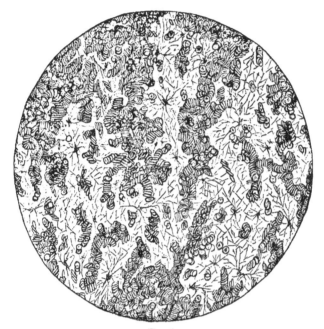

Fɪɢ. 1.

Fɪɢ. 2.

Fig. 1. — Blood in fibrous consumption.
Fig. 2. — Blood in rheumatism.

PLATE XIV.

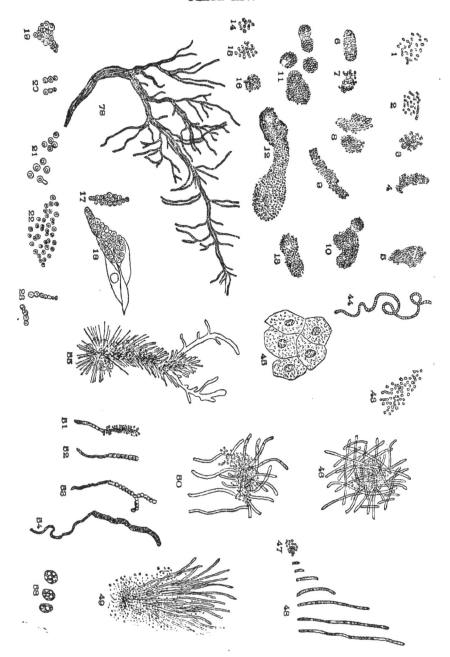

Figs. 1–16. — Spores of acid yeasts in the expectoration of consumption.

Figs. 17, 18, 19, 20, 21, 22, and 23. — Spores of a yeast vegetation developing in the skin, in tubercular consumption.

Figs. 43, 46, and 49. — Spores and filaments of leptothrix, found in the sputa of consumption.

Figs. 50, 51, 52, 53, 54, and 55. — Vegetations found in the sputa of tubercular consumption.

Fig. 78. — Shreds of breaking-down connective tissue found in the sputa of the last stage of consumption.

PLATE XV.

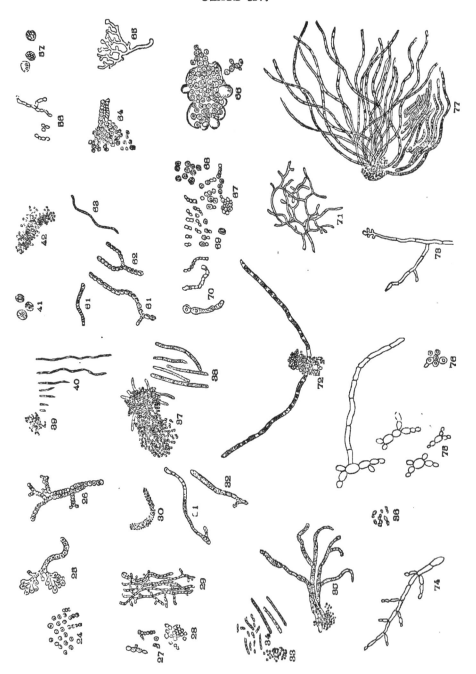

Figs 24, 66, 67, 68, and 76. — Spores of a yeast vegetation developing in the skin in tubercular
consumption, in its later stages.

Figs. 25, 26, 27, 28, 29, 30, 31, 32, 33, 34, 35, 36, 37, 38, 39, 40, 42, 56, 57, 61, 62, 63, 64, 70,
71, 72, 73, 74, 75, and 77. — Vegetations in the expectoration of tubercular consumption
in the last or breaking-down stage.

PLATE XVI.

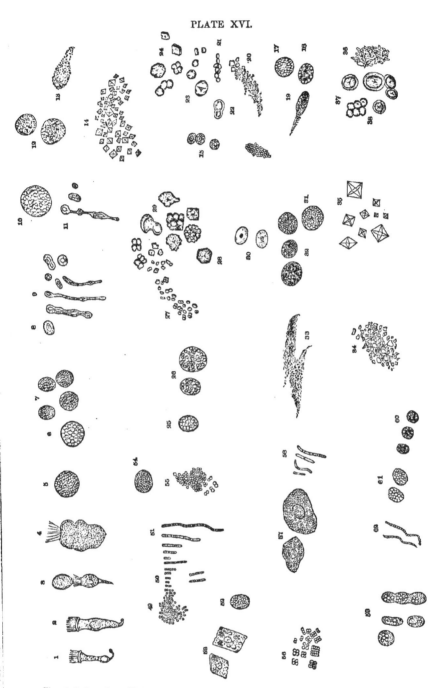

Figs. 1, 2, 3, and 4. Various appearances of cells of ciliated epithelia as expectorated in asthma. — Figs. 5, 6, 7, 10, 12, 13, 17, 18, 19, 25, 26, 31, 32, and 54. Various appearances of the giant cells expectorated in asthma. — Figs. 8, 9, and 11. Albuminoid matter (undergoing amœboid changes) escaped from the giant cells. — Figs. 14, 20, 21, 22, 23, 24, 27, 28, 29, 34, 35, 36, 37, and 38. Crystals and calculi found in expectorations of asthma. — Figs. 49, 50, 51, 55, 56, 58, and 62. Appearance of some of the vegetations developing in the sputa of asthma.

PLATE XVII.

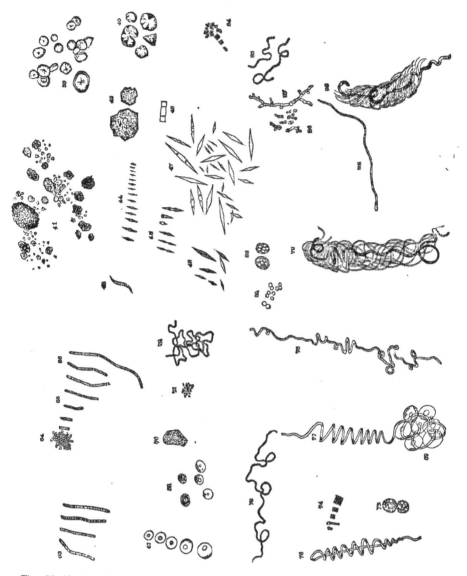

Figs. 39, 40, 41, and 42. — Calculi coughed up in gravel of the lungs, or asthma.

Figs. 44, 45, 46, and 47. — Double fusiform crystals in asthmatic expectoration.

Fig. 48. — Spore of species of fucidium.

Figs. 63, 64, 65, 66, 71, 72, 73, 74, 82, 83, 84, 85, 86, 87, and 88. — Various vegetations found in sputa of asthma.

Figs. 76, 77, 78, 79, and 80. — Species of spirulina developing in the air cells in asthma.

PLATE XVIII.

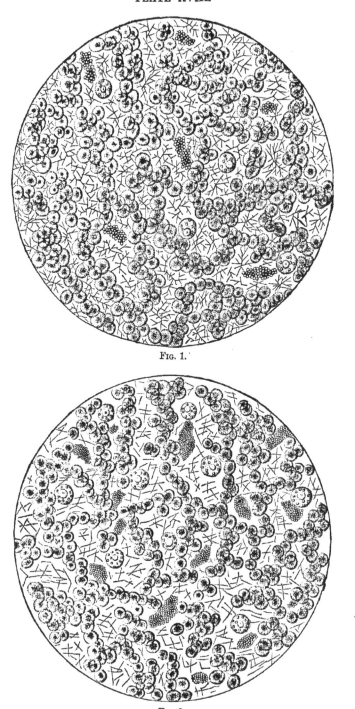

Fig. 1.

Fig. 2.

Figs. 1 and 2. — Appearance and condition of blood in swine when they have died of
tubercular consumption and consumption of bowels.

PLATE XIX.

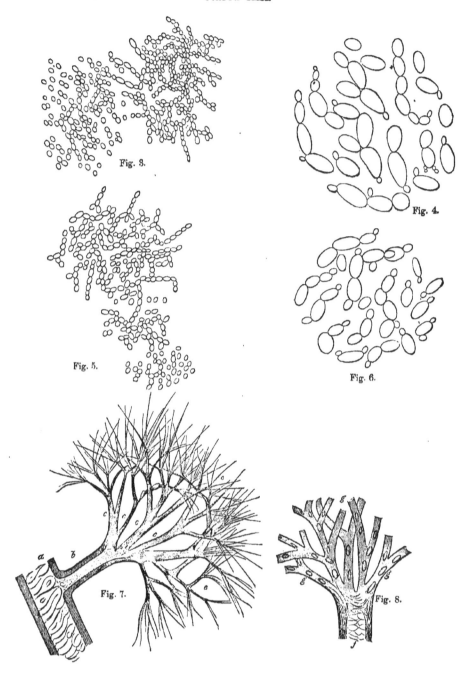

Fig. 3.

Fig. 4.

Fig. 5.

Fig. 6.

Fig. 7.

Fig. 8.

INDEX.

---

histology; organs and tissues — and cause, is the first step in handling disease, 167.
Determination of author to discover the causes of disease, iv.
Devils, imaginary sight of, 195.
Diabetes mellitus, 21, 86.
caused by a stasis in liver, 39.
caused by feeding, 208.
caused by reckless feeding, 130.
cure consists in cutting off all foods which make sugar, 132.
only hope is in soulful determination, 130.
the lobules of the liver make more sugar than is needed, 131.
treatment of, 127.
Diagnosis of a case of consumption, microscopical, 167.
valuable, by fibrin filaments, examination, 158.
Diaphragm gets vitality from cerebellum, 6.
in consumption, partially paralyzed by CO_2 absorbed from stomach, 72.
mostly paralyzed, 220.
Diarrhœa, 197, 198.
aggravated by astringents while fermenting food is kept up, 148.
from army biscuit diet, 23, 203, 212.
chronic, not amenable to ordinary treatment, 198.
from baked beans diet, 185, 186.
profuse, 187.
from using salt meats, 149.
oatmeal diet, 195, 196.
old cases of, grow fat, 150.
on army biscuit diet, not as liable to come when soldiers are active, 198.
yeasts, 221.
Did not want to get up; oatmeal diet, 194.
Diet during nursing, 296.
healthy, causes catarrhs to go, 109.
in fibræmia, 139.
in motherhood, 16.
in pregnancy, 295.
of armies in producing diseases, 148.
of infants after weaning, 17.
on vinegar in excess; experiments, 218.
removes the elongated folds of bowels, 147.
Digestive apparatus, a yeast-pot in consumption, 37.
organs becoming a well-established apparatus for developing yeasts, culminating in fatty degeneration, 142.
organs in each class of animals determine its natural food, 294.
Digitaline, 113.
Diluted, highly, and stuffed food might produce hog-cholera, 284.
Dinner, 222.
Diphtheria germs worked up, 1862, vi.
Diphtheritic exudation, 58.
Diplopia from oatmeal diet, 195.
Directions to obtain the blood for microscopical examination, 152.
Discharges in acute stage of consumption of the bowels and chronic diarrhœa, 52.
Discovery of the cause of consumption of the

lungs and bowels, and thrombosis, by experiments on swine, 224.
Disease cured by special feeding, 21.
is not confined to the body, 177.
proceeds along the line of least resistance, 25.
should be detected in embryo by the physician, 167.
Diseases arising from unhealthy alimentation, 21.
due to civilization, 14.
mostly based on violation of dietetic laws, 207.
the terrible outcome of defective and unhealthy feeding, save those from parasites, poisons, and injuries, 294.
Disinclination to move, seventh day army biscuit diet, 199.
Disinclined to exertion on oatmeal diet, 193.
to move about or talk, oatmeal diet, 195.
Disposed to lie down, oatmeal diet, 194.
Distention from army biscuit diet, 194.
of bowels great on twelfth day, army biscuit diet, 200.
Distillers thought hog-cholera contagious, and practiced isolation uselessly, 284.
Distillery of Henry Smith, 224.
Distress a sign of meat dyspepsia, 209.
Divine, the, how to receive and manifest like nature, 204.
Dizziness, disappears, oatmeal diet, 196.
in fibræmia, 139.
after diarrhœa, 203.
relieved, 223.
Dizzy, army biscuit diet, 199.
cured by meat-eating, 187.
from baked beans diet, 185, 186.
from oatmeal diet, 194, 195.
relieved after diarrhœa, 203.
sixteenth day, 201–203.
Does not like to be disturbed, 195.
Door found ajar, v.
Downward working of colds, 108.
Drags feet on walking, army biscuit diet, 203.
Drawbacks, 176.
cause of, in ethical relations of physician and patient, 177.
Drawings have been made of the different blood morphologies, iv, 152.
Draw the lines tightly when lapses occur, 169.
Dreaming, army biscuit diet, seventh day, 199.
Dreams, troubled, army biscuit diet, sixth day, 199.
Drinks and foods have to do with chronic ailments, 2.
in Bright's disease, 122.
in consumption, 92.
in diabetes, 127.
in fibræmia, 139, 140.
in fibrosis and locomotor ataxy, ovarian tumors, etc., 135.
Drives, 125, 128, 137.
Driving, 140.
Dropsy, 150.
in fibræmia, 141.
Drunk, feels, from baked beans diet, 185, 186.

Vinegar yeast, in blood, 219 ; increasing, 220, 221.
in blood, 104 out of 104 cases, 285.
Virchow, 61, 66.
Viscid mucus, 148.
Vision impaired, 213.
Vis medicatrix naturæ, 285.
Vital energy, a stock in trade for life, 10.
every pound should be utilized, 10.
expended injudiciously, 11.
how to accumulate, 180.
its judicious use needful, 5.
limited, 10.
may be wasted, 9, 10.
not controlled by will power, 10.
one of two great factors in life, 5.
one should economically increase and store it, 9.
saved by contemplation, 180.
should be used for organic uses and necessities, 174.
thrown away recklessly by athletes, 10.
thrown away recklessly by base-ball players, health lift, etc., 11.
uselessly expended, 5.
Vital fact for man, that nearly all our diseases come from food, 294.
Voice weak and husky, 78, 195.
weak and impaired, 212.
Vomiting, 9.
Voracious, 213.

WAIT, 299.
Wakeful, 219.
Wakeful and uneasy all night, oatmeal diet, 194 ; army biscuit diet, sixteenth day, nineteenth day, 201.
army biscuit diet, twentieth day, 202.
Wakefulness common in fibræmia, 139.
due to a tendency to reversed action, 9.
Wakes in fright, with heart beating violently, oatmeal diet, 195.
Walk unsteady on baked beans diet, 186.
Walks, 125, 128.
with difficulty, twenty-second day, army biscuit diet, 202 ; easier, 204.
with difficulty on baked beans diet, 186, 187.
Wandering pains on oatmeal diet, 193.
Want of knowledge as to the causes of disease, iii.
Warts, 67.
Washing out a case of consumption, 168.
Water, 172, 198.
cold, 95.
fennel seed, 113.
hot, 94, 97, 122, 127, 135, 140, 144, 168.
ice, bad, 95.
lukewarm, vomits, 96.
in Swiss mountains not the cause of goitre, 216.
We all expend force too much in the cerebrum, 8.
We are two thirds carnivorous and one third herbivorous by structure, 297.
We should live in the cerebellum, etc., more, 8.
We should live less in the garret of our house and more in the kitchen, 8, 9.

Weak and languid, army biscuit diet, eighteenth day, 201.
heart, 208.
on baked beans diet, 186, 187.
Weakest organ the first victim of disease, 24.
Weakness, 208.
army biscuit diet, 202.
muscular, in fatty degeneration, 143.
Weaning should take place from twelfth to eighteenth month, 297.
Weight, loss of, under treatment, need excite no apprehension, 136.
of men put on army biscuit diet, 199.
of six men put on baked beans and coffee, 184 ; weight lost, 188.
of six hundred and twenty-four hogs ranging each from one hundred to three hundred pounds, 231.
Well, 196.
Wet-nurse, 297.
Wheat, cracked, one part to four or six, 98.
in Bright's disease, 123.
in diabetes, 128.
Wheaten grits can be fed exclusively forty to fifty days, 207.
Whiskey, 174, 198.
distillery slop feeding to hogs prepared author for feeding man, 218.
Whole nature, moral and physical, must be brought to the task, 178.
Wild cherry, 171.
Wild cherry bark, 113.
Will-power not a balance-wheel nor a safety-valve to check waste of nerve-force, 5.
Wind in stomach and bowels on oatmeal diet, 193.
Wing & Smith's hog-pens, 224.
Wisdom displayed by fatty degeneration process, 142.
Witch hazel, 171.
fluid extract of, 93.
Wobbled on baked beans diet, 187.
Women, the most beautiful, have goitre, 217.
Woodcock, 122.
Worcestershire sauce, 98, 122, 127, 135, 140.
Work should be done for its own integral sake, 183.
"Work that could not be done with kid gloves," hog cholera studies, v.
Work without faith is dead, 177.
Worries, senseless, weaken the mind, 182.
Worry, a cause of sloughing of intestines, 174.
controlled by stopping causes and using healthy mental efforts, 6.
due to insane sympathetic nerves, 5.
how to get relief from, 7 ; rationale of process, 7.
Worrying, an outward expression of disease, 6.
Wrong impression as to blood examination, 156.
Wrong-doing must cease before we can cure disease, 126.

YEARS, three, it may take to cure asthma, consumption, 113 ; fibrous diseases, 136.

1,000,000 Books

are available to read at

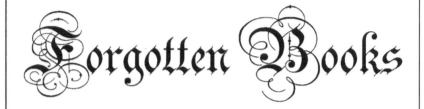

---◆---

www.ForgottenBooks.com

---◆---

Read online
Download PDF
Purchase in print

ISBN 978-0-282-77287-1
PIBN 10864286